DEPARTMENT OF PAEDIATRIC SURGERY
UNIVERSITY HOSPITAL
QUEEN'S MEDICAL CENTRE
NOTTINGHAM

# Surgery for Hirschsprung's Disease

General Editor, Wolfe Surgical Atlases:
William F. Walker, DSc, ChM, FRCS (Edin. and
England), FRS (Edin.).

Single Surgical Procedures 21

A Colour Atlas of

# Surgery for Hirschsprung's Disease

## H. Homewood Nixon

MA, MB, B.Chir, FRCS(Eng), FACS(Hon), FAAP(Hon)
*Honorary Consulting Surgeon,
The Hospital for Sick Children
Great Ormond Street, London
and St Mary's Hospital, London
and Honorary Senior Lecturer in
Surgery, Institute of Child Health,
University of London*

(Photography by Ray Lunnon, M.Phil,
FBIPP, FRPS, AIMBI, Director, Department
of Medical Illustration, Hospital for Sick
Children, Great Ormond Street, London).

Copyright © H. Homewood Nixon, 1985
Published by Wolfe Medical Publications Ltd, 1985
Printed by Royal Smeets Offset b.v.,
Weert, Netherlands
ISBN 0 7234 1011 9

This book is one of the titles in the series of
Wolfe Single Surgical Procedures, a series which
will eventually cover some 200 titles.

If you wish to be kept informed of new
additions to the series and receive details of our
other titles, please write to
Wolfe Medical Publications Ltd, Wolfe House,
3 Conway Street, London W1P 6HE.

# Contents

# Acknowledgements

I am greatly indebted to my colleagues, past and present, for their many informal discussions which contribute so much to a surgical career. I am particularly indebted to Mr Ray Lunnon (Figures **9, 11–13, 15–19, 21–25, 27–38, 41, 42, 44–55, 58, 65, 66, 75, 76**) for his outstandingly expert photography which made the book possible; also to Mrs Gillian Oliver for the excellent diagrams and to Miss Lilian Haylock for her efficient and patient production of the typescript.

# Introduction

Although this is an atlas of the definitive surgery for Hirschsprung's disease, it is necessary to make some more general comments on the disease itself to clarify the range of clinical and pathological entities under discussion, and hence the indications for and timing of the procedures, before describing the operations in detail.

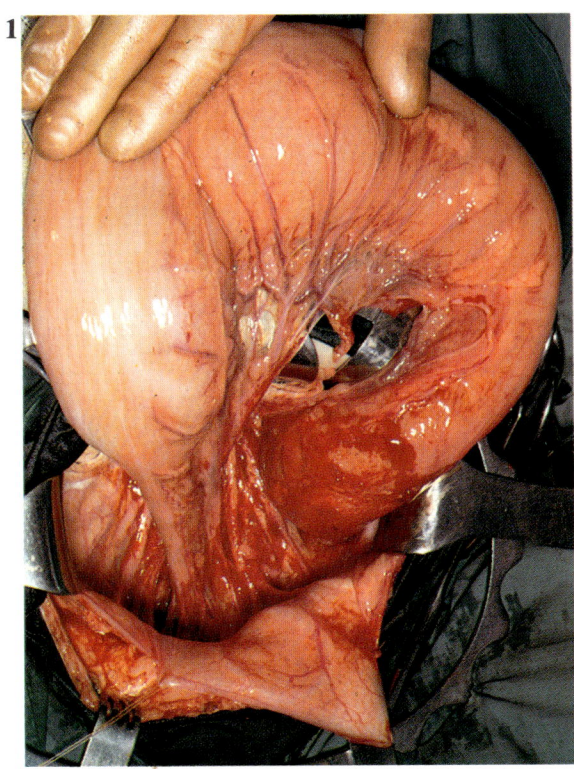

**1** 'Classical' megacolon and unexpanded (*not necessarily narrow*) rectum.

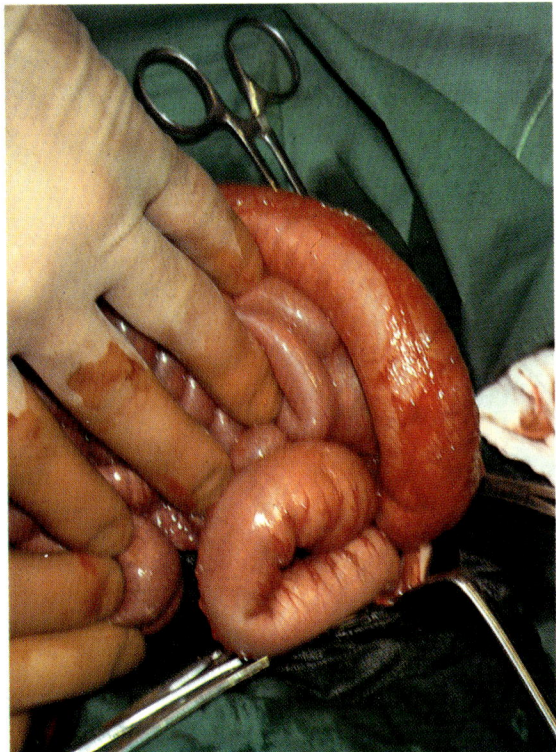

**2** Less marked but clearly recognisable transition from megacolon to unexpanded aganglionic rectum in a newborn.

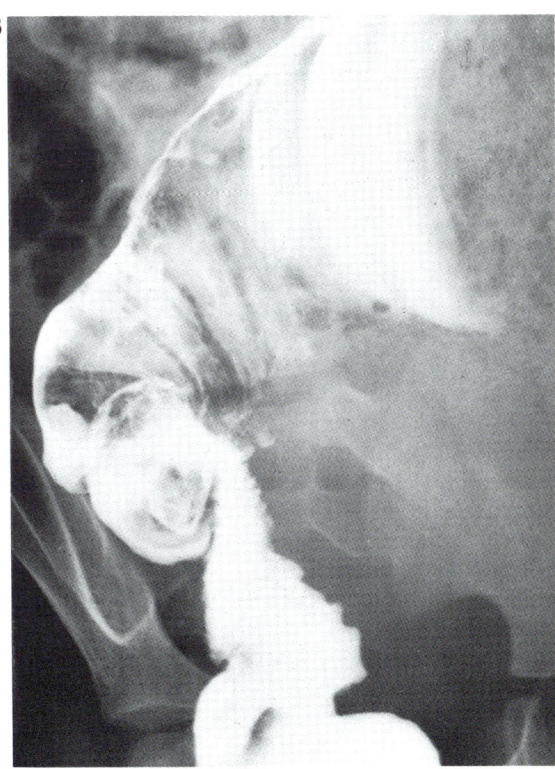

**3** Barium enema demonstration of the crucial 'cone' of narrowing from the megacolon to the unexpanded aganglionic rectum.

Hirschsprung's disease can be defined as congenital distal intestinal aganglionosis. (There are other causes of megacolon and there are rare other neuropathies which will not be considered here (Nixon and Lake, 1982).)

Hirschsprung's disease presents a wide spectrum from chronic constipation to acute complete neonatal intestinal obstruction. Passage of meconium is delayed beyond the first 24 hours of life in 90 per cent but other neonatal symptoms may be transient or even, very rarely, absent. Nevertheless, in the typical case it is the early onset of the bowel symptoms which will give rise to the clinical suspicion of the disease and these will be obstructive rather than merely of constipation.

The author has treated 310 children at Great Ormond Street from 1949 to 1977 (Frank and Nixon) and over that period a remarkable change in presentation had occurred. Now we see even more neonatal and early infant patients than 'classical cases' in older children with gross wasting and vast abdominal girth. The incidence in the population has seemed to rise as the clinically severe neonatal instances have been recognised, and particularly those with the potentially fatal enterocolitis which caused a paradoxical presentation with distension but also with 'spurious diarrhoea', commonly in the past leading to a disastrous misdiagnosis of gastro-enteritis (Table 1).

Table 2 gives the 'classical' distinguishing factors from the acquired megacolon of habitual constipation. Because rectal suction biopsy is now a safe and reliable diagnostic measure (Noblett, 1969; Lake et al, 1978) one should now anticipate that most cases will be diagnosed in early infancy. (It should be noted that in the cases with complications reported by Rees et al, (1983) in none had the technique described by Noblett been followed.) This early diagnosis is very important because the complication of enterocolitis remains the commonest cause of death in Hirschsprung's disease. So it will be usual now for the patient to present for the definitive operation in infancy with a colostomy having already been performed. Milder cases and those who have avoided enterocolitis will still present later in a significant proportion.

---

**Table 1. Overall mortality of Hirschsprung's disease.**

1949 to 1977

n = 310

41 Died = 13%

Pre-colostomy      3 = 1%

Post-colostomy  20 = 6.5%

Post-pullthrough 18 = 6%

Early 13              Late 5*

4.5%                     1.5%

*One as late as 8 years after successful operation with no residual symptoms. (Frank and Nixon 1979.)

---

**Table 2. Typical clinical pictures.**

|  | Hirschsprung's Disease | Rectal Inertia |
|---|---|---|
| Onset | Neonatal | 'Training' period |
| Constipation | + | + |
| Distension | + | − |
| Peristalsis | + + | − |
| Rectum | Empty | Loaded |
| Soiling | − | + |
| General health | → Poor | Reasonable |
| Risk to life | High | Negligible |

**4** The Swenson prolapse technique.

**5** The Duhamel retrorectal transanal technique.

**6** The Soave non-sutured endorectal technique.

**7** The Denda/Scott Boley sutured endorectal technique.

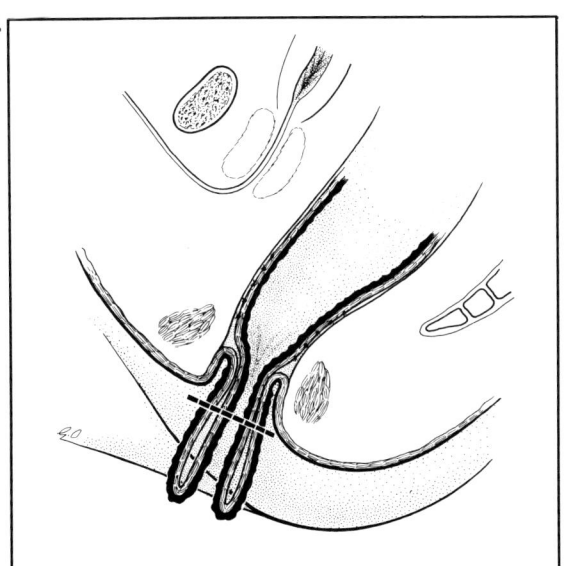

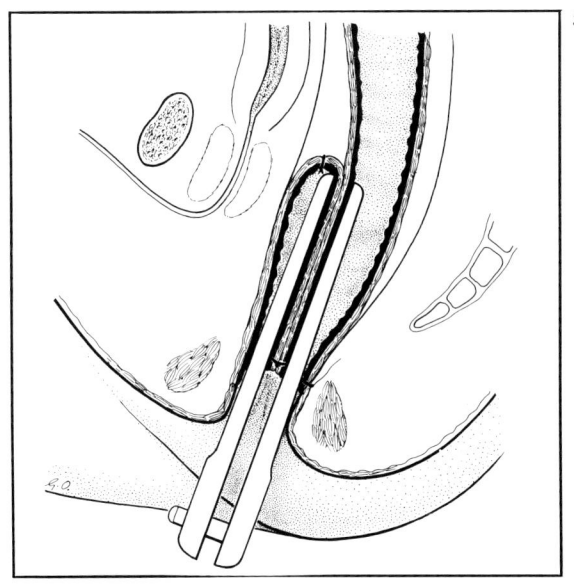

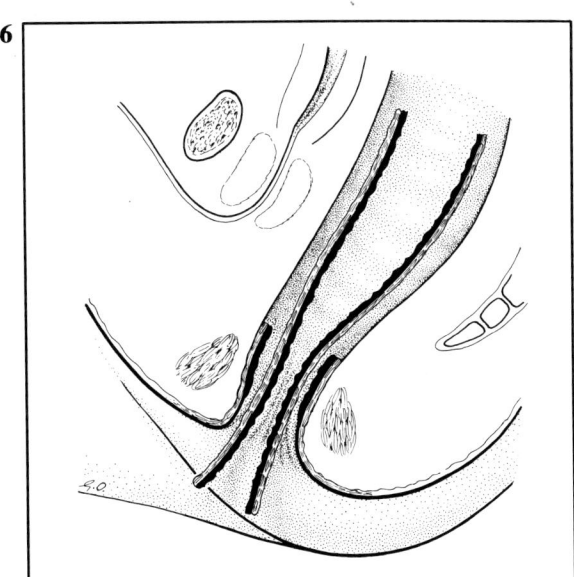

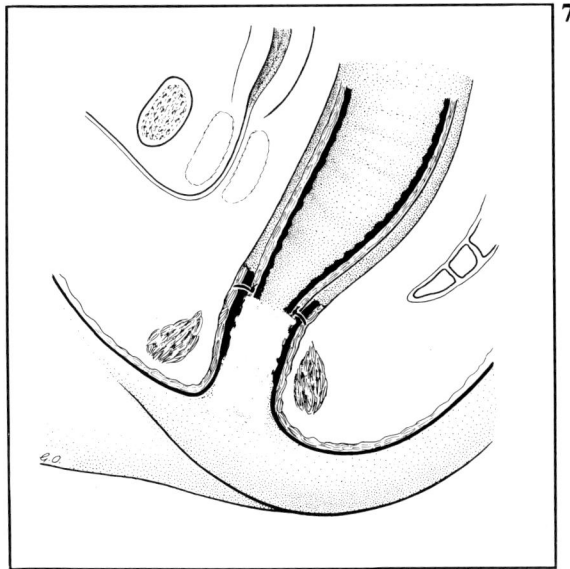

The object of the definitive operation is to resect or bypass the abnormal segment of distal bowel. There are three main techniques of operation to achieve this. Rectosigmoidectomy by a prolapse and excision manoeuvre, successfully introduced by Swenson in 1948 and modified (Swenson 1964), is the oldest of these established procedures (**4**). The retrorectal transanal operation, devised by Duhamel (1960), is an alternative which avoids a tedious (though not really difficult) dissection below the pelvic floor (**5**). The endorectal technique is the third of the established methods and is an application of the mucosal stripping technique recommended by Ravitch and Sabiston (1947) for polyposis and ulcerative colitis. Soave (1966) introduced a non-suture anastomotic technique which had the advantage of avoiding the need for covering colostomy but the disadvantage of requiring postoperative dilatations (**6**). Denda in Japan and Scott Boley in America independently described a sutured modification which should not need postoperative dilatations (**7**).

Although many surgeons carry out these techniques without a covering colostomy when a suitably healthy and well-prepared patient presents, yet my own experience has convinced me that complications though rare can be so severe as to risk continence or even life, so that I do not personally consider this to be in general justified except in the staged endorectal techniques which really amount to a perineal colostomy after the first stage.

An alternative group of operations involves resection of the bowel only down to the pelvic floor as in an anterior resection, but accompanying this with either forcible dilatation of the sphincter below or a formal myectomy. This has been widely used by Professor Rehbein and his followers (Rehbein 1964) but as it may require repeated postoperative dilatation, and as the other techniques had shown their worth, I have no personal experience of it.

The usual patient will, therefore, present with an aganglionic segment involving the rectum and the lower sigmoid colon, having a colostomy already present. I find it convenient to operate when the baby is established and gaining weight at three to six months of age, although there is no bar to earlier definitive operation in the correct paediatric surgical setting. There appears to be no special magic in waiting for either the first birthday or a weight of 18lb (8.5 kilos) as has often been recommended. It is indeed easier to operate in the shallow pelvis of the young infant provided that one has the correct equipment and support.

## Special circumstances

The wide clinical spectrum of the disease does produce special considerations in individual instances which may be as follows.

**The segment** The segment may be shorter, only involving part of the rectum. This gives no clinical problem in management except in the so-called ultra short segment, which is perhaps better called 'anal achalasia' in which only anal dilatation or myectomy (Lynn, 1968) may be necessary, avoiding the need for a major surgical procedure. Diagnosis may have to depend on anorectal manometry if the segment is so short that only the internal sphincter lacks its intrinsic innervation.

Longer segments also occur. If the segment reaches above the sigmoid colon then an extended colonic resection is required. If it is necessary to bring down the right colon to the anus, the preferred technique is to rotate the mesenteric pedicle 180 degrees to bring down the colon on the right side, rather than trying to draw it round in a more natural position.

Total colonic aganglionosis occurs in about four per cent of patients. Because there is then no colonic reservoir and the ileum has to be brought down, the Duhamel procedure which preserves the rectal reservoir is preferred because it gives an easier postoperative course, although the other techniques can be satisfactory in the long run after an initial period of unpleasantly frequent stooling. I believe that it is more important to leave the child with ileostomy for at least three months to 'colonise' the bowel before doing the pullthrough, than to attempt to construct a particularly large reservoir by greatly extending the side-to-side junction of the Duhamel operation in order to maintain adequate fluid balance.

An even rarer variant is that in which there is total colonic involvement plus a significant extent of the ileum. In such a case a Duhamel type resection with a longer retained segment of rectum and lower sigmoid would be advisable. The extreme procedure described by Lester Martin (1972) of side-to-side anastomosis of the small intestine to almost the complete length of the colon has had problems with stasis in other hands. A technique of lateral anastomosis of the right colon to the ileum proximal to the ileostomy, followed by a combined pullthrough of these structures with the right colon then becoming a 'free graft' vascularised from the ileum has recently been described (Kimura *et al*, 1981).

Fortunately, it is even more rare for the aganglionosis to involve the entire small gut as well as the large intestine, because this type is not only fatal but is very prone to familial recurrence.

There has been considerable scepticism about the genuine existence of skip segments, in which areas of normal innervation intervene between aganglionic segments above and below. Although extremely rare it does seem that an occasional genuine case exists. In an experience of about 400 cases the nearest I have seen to this condition is a patchy aganglionosis which I think might equally have been described as a very long transition zone. Another rarity is the presence of hyperganglionosis proximal to the aganglionic segment (Puri *et al*, 1977),

**Malnutrition** Attempts to 'tide the baby over' with rectal irrigations and aperients may have been unsuccessful in maintaining adequate nutrition. In such a case preliminary colostomy and a period of about three months to regain good general condition are advisable.

**Gross megacolon** Delayed treatment may also have allowed such a gross megacolon to develop that to perform satisfactory anastomosis one would require at that time to resect a considerable proportion of normally innervated bowel above the aganglionic segment or to taper it. Again, a colostomy for three months will give the opportunity for this proximal bowel to contract down to a more manageable size.

**Enterocolitis** This is the most serious of the special circumstances, because, as has already been said, enterocolitis is the commonest cause of death in Hirschsprung's disease and is particularly fatal in the first two months of life. Paradoxically the child presents with a 'spurious diarrhoea' in addition to abdominal distension and probably vomiting. Unlike the necrotising enterocolitis more commonly seen in premature babies, pneumatosis is extremely rare but investigations (Thomas *et al*, 1982) have shown that clostridium difficile is involved in some though not in all the cases. This is important because in such cases oral vancomycin may be dramatically successful in relieving the symptoms. Nevertheless, one must not fail to carry out the more non-specific management, deflating the abdomen by saline irrigations, then proceeding to colostomy. This is safer than an immediate colostomy which is sometimes followed a few hours later by an intense vasomotor collapse. Intravenous fluids and antibiotics are also given at this stage.

**The site of the colostomy** A right transverse colostomy is very convenient for the usual case because it can be left to cover the definitive pullthrough procedure. However, if it is carried out in the first two or three weeks of life, before the sigmoid loop has had the opportunity to enlarge and lengthen its mesentery, then it may be found that the vessels rather than the bowel itself may not be long enough to enable the bowel to be brought down to the anus without tension. Therefore, it is preferable in the neonatal period to carry out a terminal colostomy immediately above the aganglionic zone. (Indeed this is equally satisfactory in older patients – its only disadvantage being the need, in my opinion, to add a further proximal covering colostomy to the definitive operation.) I prefer to bring out the distal end of the bowel as a mucus fistula rather than dropping it back into the peritoneum, because this gives an easy approach to the rectum at the definitive operation. If the distal bowel is dropped back into the pelvis, the small intestine can sometimes form tiresome adhesions over it. This technique requires the availability of competent frozen section cover at the time of operation. If such cover is not available in a great emergency, I have found that a reasonable clinical guide seems to be that the bowel will be ganglionic 5 cm above the upper end of the cone of transition from the unexpanded bowel to the megacolon when the segment is of the usual length. If the apparent cone is proximal to the sigmoid, however, it is so likely to be a false cone lower down than the extent of ganglionic bowel that it would be safer in such an emergency to carry out a formal ileostomy.

It is most important either to have the colostomy as a formal right transverse colostomy proximal to the intended operation for the pull-through or to have it as low as possible in the ganglionic bowel. Anything in between these levels is liable to complicate mobilisation at the definitive operation, and may involve resecting more bowel than would otherwise have been necessary. The colostomy technique is also important. A formal matured colostomy should be made even in the neonate just as precisely as one would in the older patient. Stenosis of the colostomy can produce fluid and electrolyte losses akin to those of ileostomy dysfunction. Use of the skin bridge technique (Nixon, 1966) has eliminated mortality resulting from colostomy itself but has not been as successful as one hoped in avoidance of prolapse, usually of the distal loop. An end colostomy has seemed to cause the least trouble in this respect.

## Operation without preliminary colostomy

In my hands I am convinced that there is an added safety in carrying out either preoperative colostomy or a covering colostomy at the time of the operation, because the anastomosis is under the pelvic floor and does not have a serous coat to protect it. It is hence intrinsically at a greater risk for leakage. This leakage may be insignificant but even minor degrees of fibrosis around the sphincters may interfere with the finer points of continence and aganglionosis is a benign condition in a child with all life before it. Furthermore, occasionally such a leakage may cause a pelvic cellulitis which can interfere with the continence of the bladder as well as the bowel, or even a potentially fatal anaerobic septicaemia. Rare as these problems are I feel that they are so serious that they justify routine colostomy with all the techniques to be described except the non-suture or staged suture type of endorectal anastomosis (Table 3). In 1958 I independently developed an endorectal technique with a staged anastomosis which is perhaps midway between the original Soave and the Denda/Scott Boley sutured endorectal in which the results followed up to 20 years later are entirely satisfactory (8). My only reason for leaving the technique was that it did sometimes require postoperative dilatations which were potentially upsetting to the baby. Since a secondary procedure is required to trim off the excess bowel about 14 days after the definitive operation the period in hospital is not so much less than if a covering colostomy is used.

**Table 3.  Swenson operations.**

| Complications | 1949–1977: no = 155 | |
| | Colostomy cover | No cover |
| --- | --- | --- |
| | n = 46 | n = 109 |
| Enterocolitis | 6 (13%) | 14 (13%) |
| Peritonitis | 0 | 8 (7%) |
| Bowel necrosis | 1 (2%) | 8 (7%) |
| Major leak | 0 | 16 (15%) |
| Major stricture | 0 | 10 (9%) |
| Wound infection | 7 (15%) | 15 (14%) |
| Death | 1 (2%)* | 12 (11%) |

*(Patient with Down's syndrome, renal and cardiac lesions.)

So while I now use the neat Stapler Duhamel procedure widely, I must confess that the results of the Swenson or Endorectal procedures have been similarly successful (Table 4). My practice now includes a number of patients referred after unsuccessful surgery elsewhere; in these circumstances it is useful to be familiar with the different techniques so as to be able to select a suitable one depending on the complications resulting from the previous operations. Otherwise, there need be no hesitation in choosing the technique which appeals to the individual, who will be wise to develop experience in that method rather than trying his hand too widely in the different operations. **Each one will need careful attention to every detail to avoid trouble.**

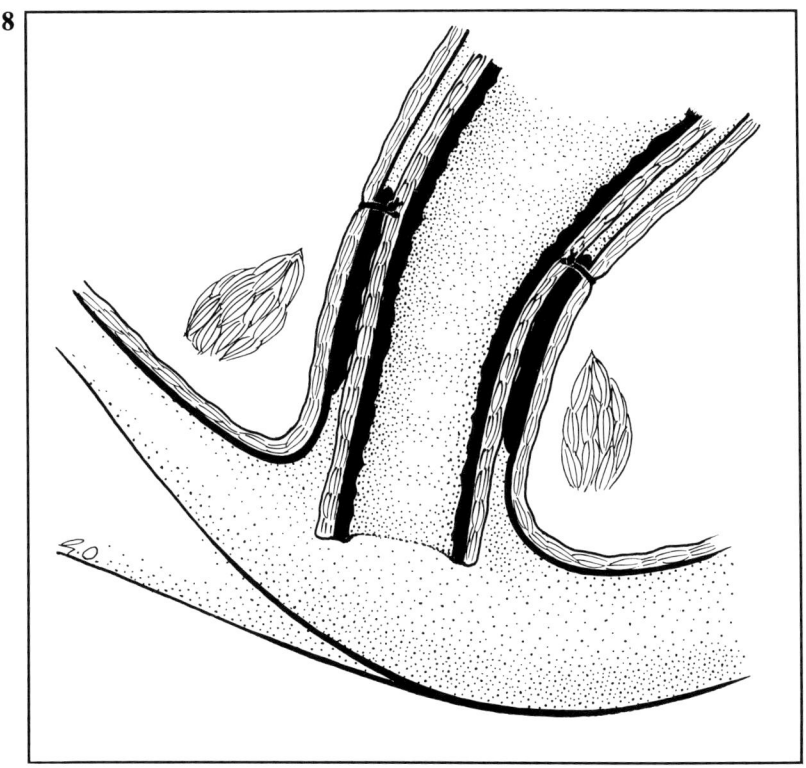

8

**8    Author's staged anastomosis endorectal technique.**

**Table 4. Comparison of Swenson, Duhamel, Soave type operations.** 1967–72: 107 operated: 62 with comparable work-up assessed

|  | Swenson | Duhamel | Soave |
|---|---|---|---|
| Number | 21 | 21 | 20 |
| Diagnosed at | 2 months–9 years | 2 months–8 years | 2 months–7 years |
| Average age at resection | 9 months | 6 months | 6 months |
| Length of gut resected<br>– Mean<br>– Range | 12 cm<br>5–29 cm | 10 cm<br>6.5–28 cm | 16.5 cm<br>10–24 cm |
| Enterocolitis | 10 | 7 | 3 |
| Late deaths from enterocolitis | 3 | 2 | 1 |
| Early postoperative deaths | 0 | 0 | 0 |
| Constipation | 13 | 6 | 1 |
| Obstructive symptoms | 7 | 3 | 2 |
| Average frequency of stooling | 3rd day | every day | >1 motion/day |
| *Fully potty trained 2½ years after op. | 6 | 10 | 8 |
| GU Problems | 0 | 0 | 0 |
| Residual complaints | 7 soiling | None | 8 loose motions |
| Ht/Wt (Mean centile) | 55/45 | 60/50 | 70/50 |

*ALL eventually achieved control. (Khan and Nixon, 1980.)

# Preoperative preparation

The following procedures must be observed with great care during preoperative preparation.
1 Check of general condition:
  (a) clinical
  (b) full blood count
  (c) serum electrolytes
  (d) serum proteins and urinalysis
2 Saline irrigations of the distal bowel until completely empty. (Occasionally a stone-like 'mucolith' may have to be left and removed with the intermediate segment of bowel.) If there is no colostomy and this is to be set up at the time of pullthrough, a liquid non-residue diet is given for two days before operation.
3 Metronidazole and neomycin cover by mouth and into the distal loop of the colostomy, and also an intravenous injection of metronidazole with the induction of anaesthesia. The aim is to have a high tissue concentration at the time of surgery.
4 Blood is cross matched.
5 A reliable intravenous line is set up – usually by the anaesthetist at the time of induction.

# Early stages of operation

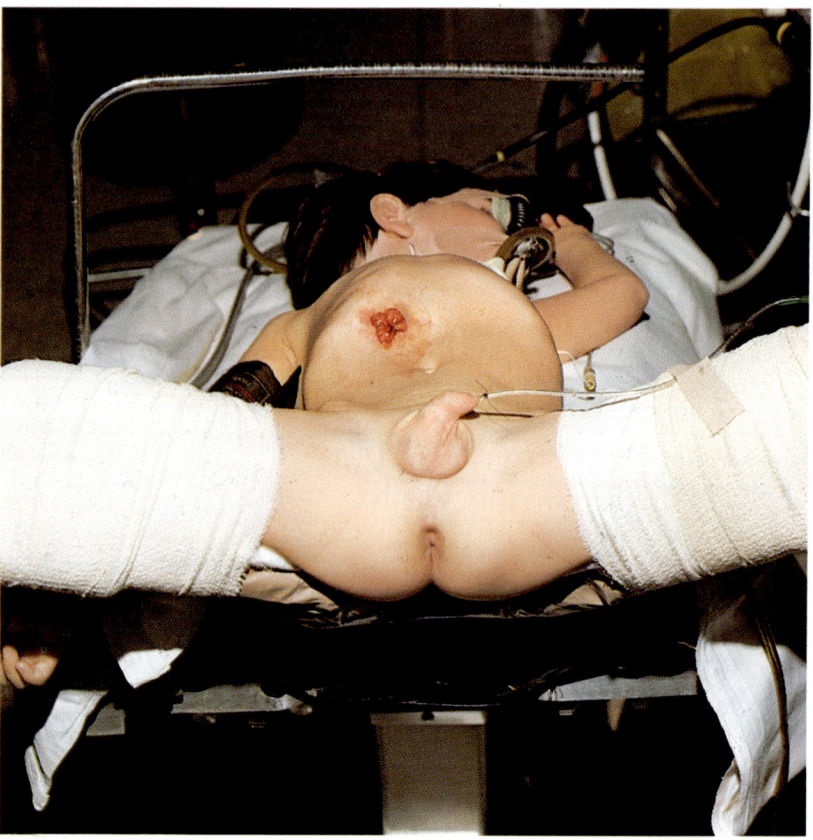

**9**

**9 To show position on table for abdominoanal operation.** Differs from that used in adult synchronous abdominoperineal operation. The pelvis is allowed to drop back over the lower end of the table and *not* tilted forward with a wedge. This gives a better view straight down the pelvis. The perineal procedure is limited to the anal canal, so there is no need to view further into the perineum from below. A urethral catheter is inserted. The colostomy, if present, is oversewn to prevent any risk of peroperative leakage. A diathermy pad is applied. A free running IV is placed, usually in the upper limb, and the anaesthetist may wish to place a central venous catheter from the neck.

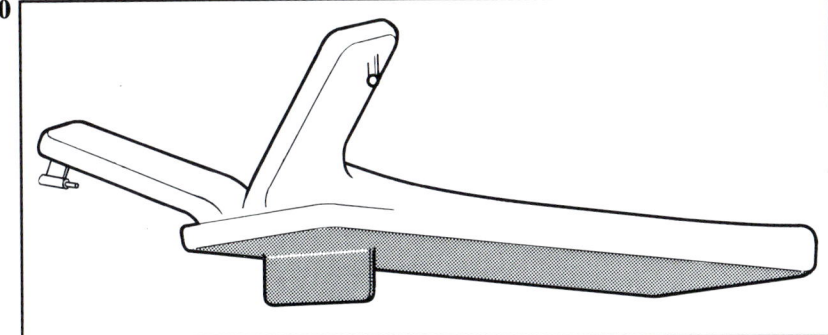

**10   This small table is strapped on to the main table when the patient is an infant.** It allows the height and tilt mechanism of the main table to be used as required, and the flange on the bottom prevents it from slipping away when the baby is head down to facilitate pelvic dissection.

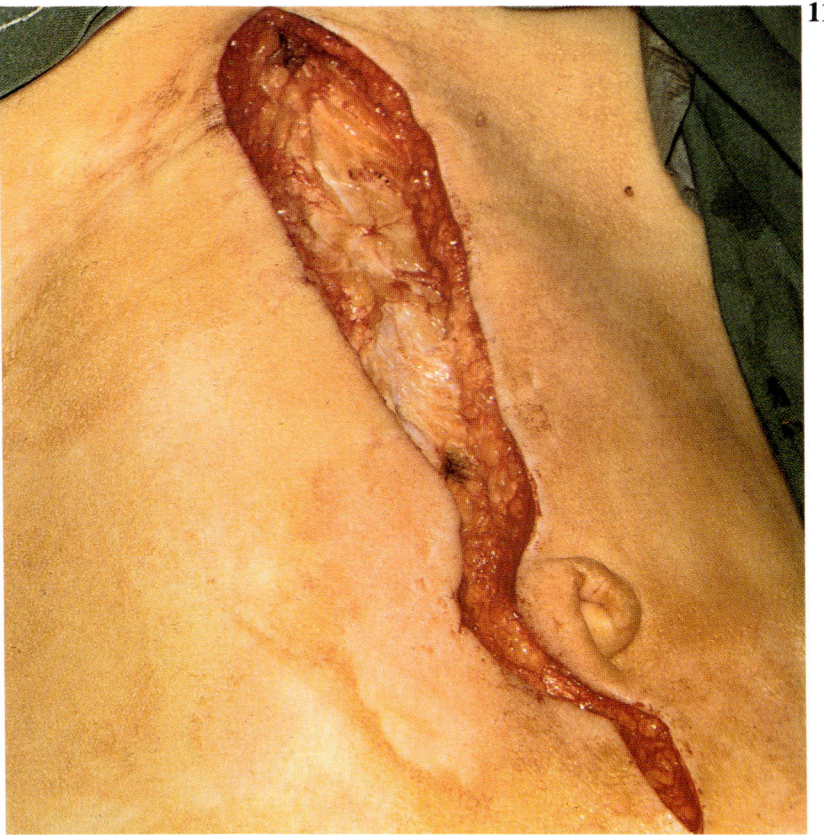

**11   A midline incision skirting the umbilicus is preferred and it must extend right down to the pubes.** (If there is an iliac colostomy, a J-shaped incision may be preferred to simplify its mobilisation.)

**12 The bladder is an abdominal organ in young children.** It must be lifted forward *out* of the abdomen. It may be necessary to divide the peritoneal incision into a Y at the lower end to achieve this result.

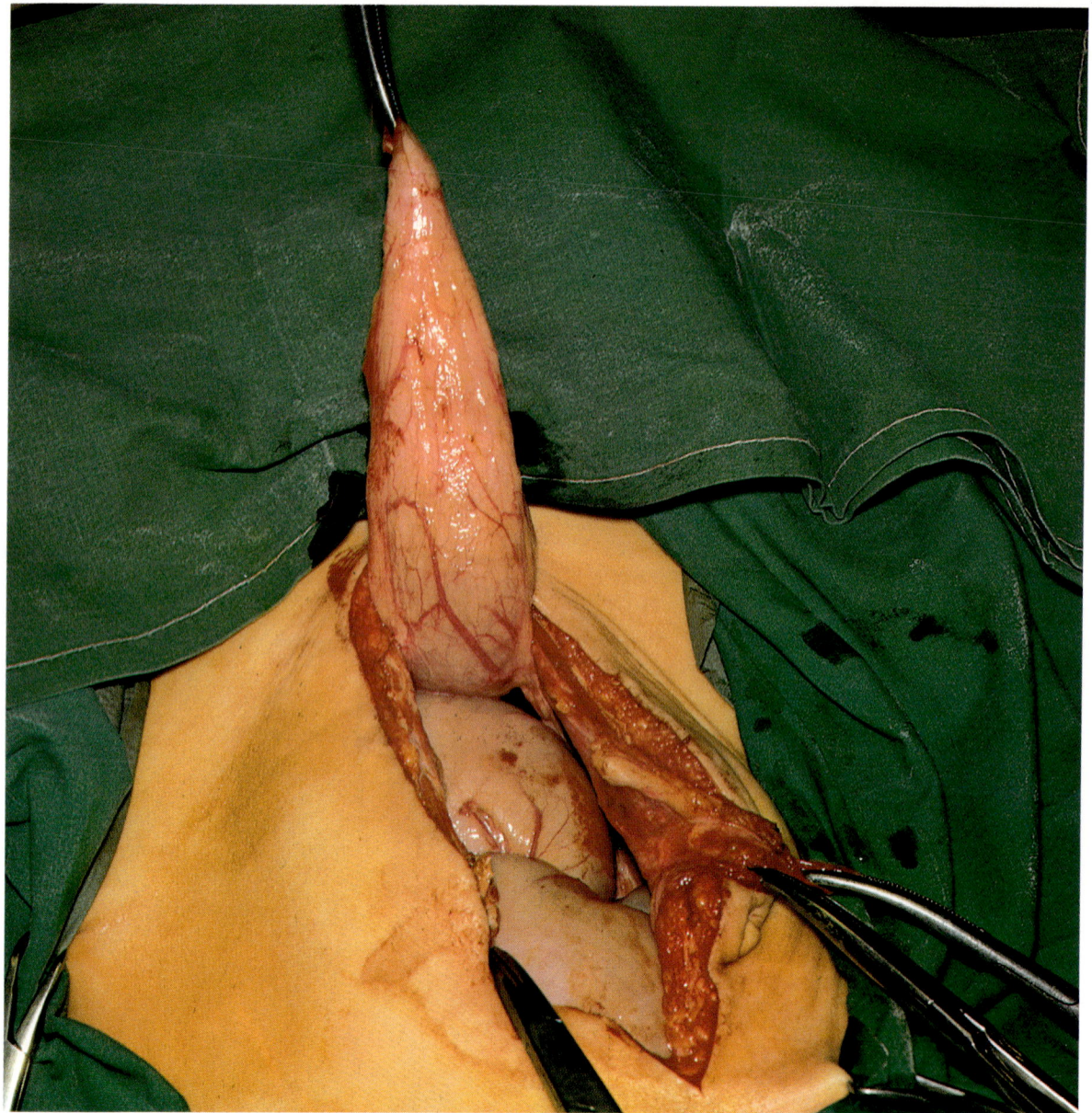

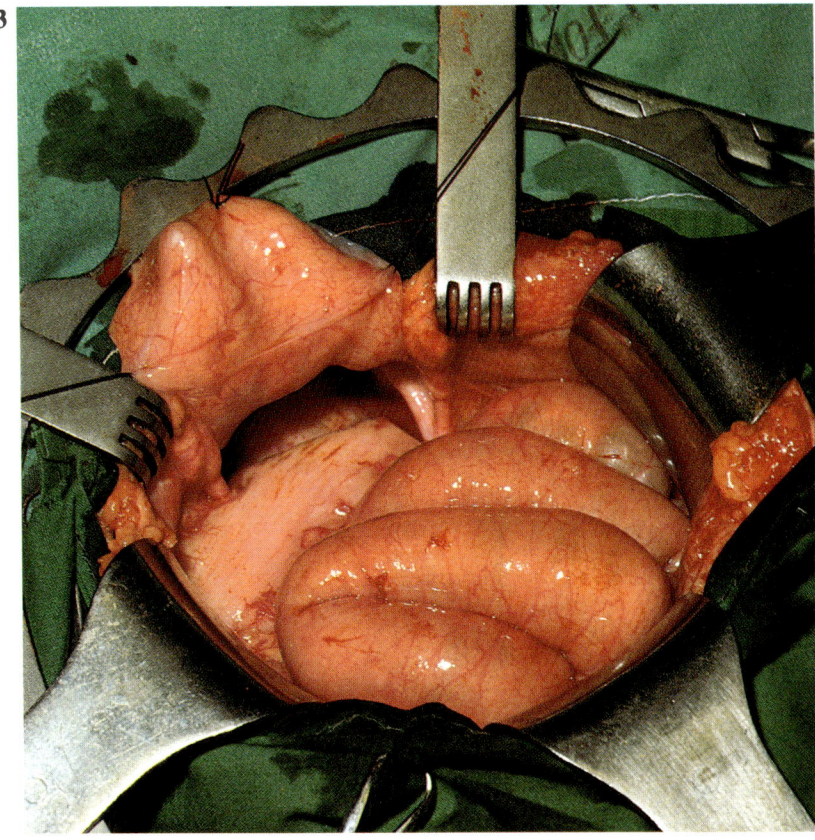

**13** Denis Browne self-retaining ring retractor inserted and bladder held out of the abdomen by stay sutures to it.

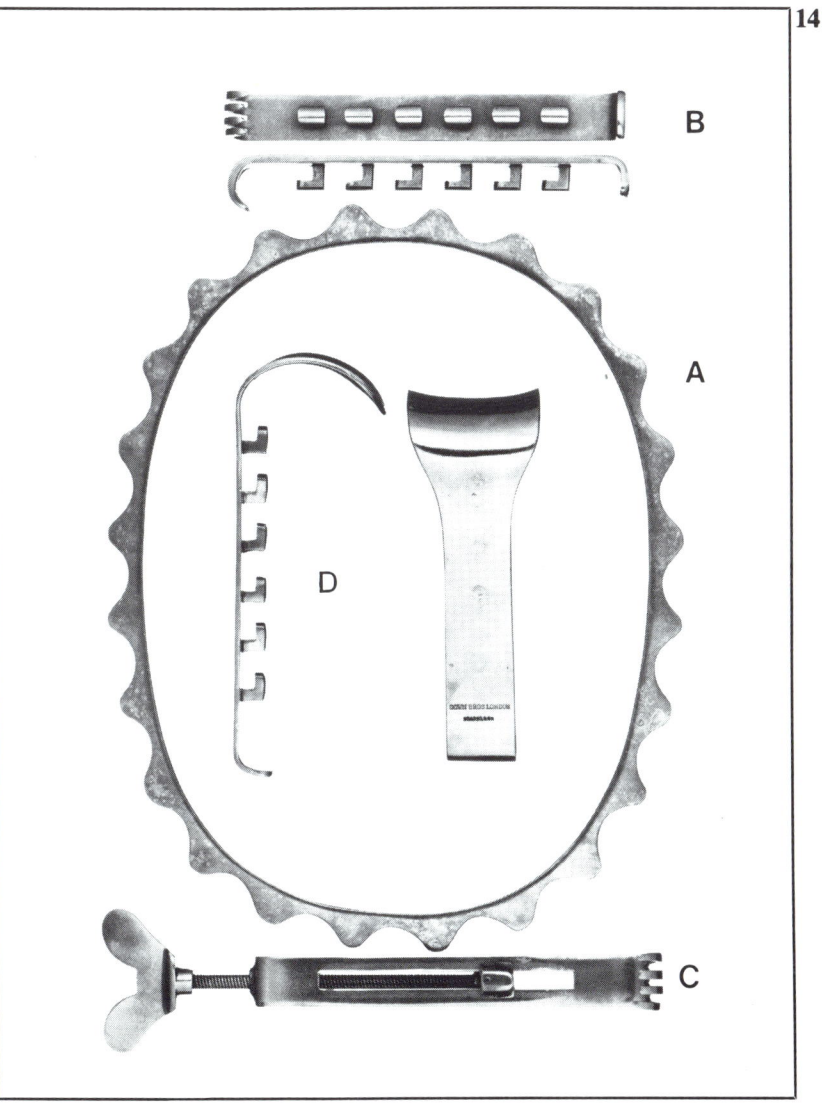

**14** The ring retractor (A), rake blades (B), screw blade (C), and abdominal blades (D).

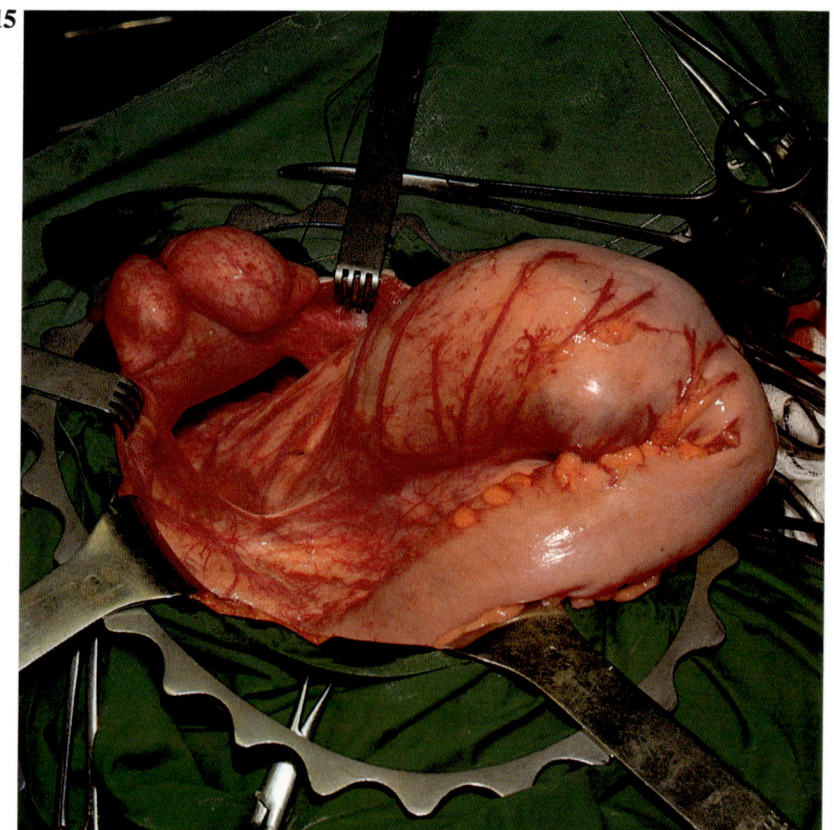

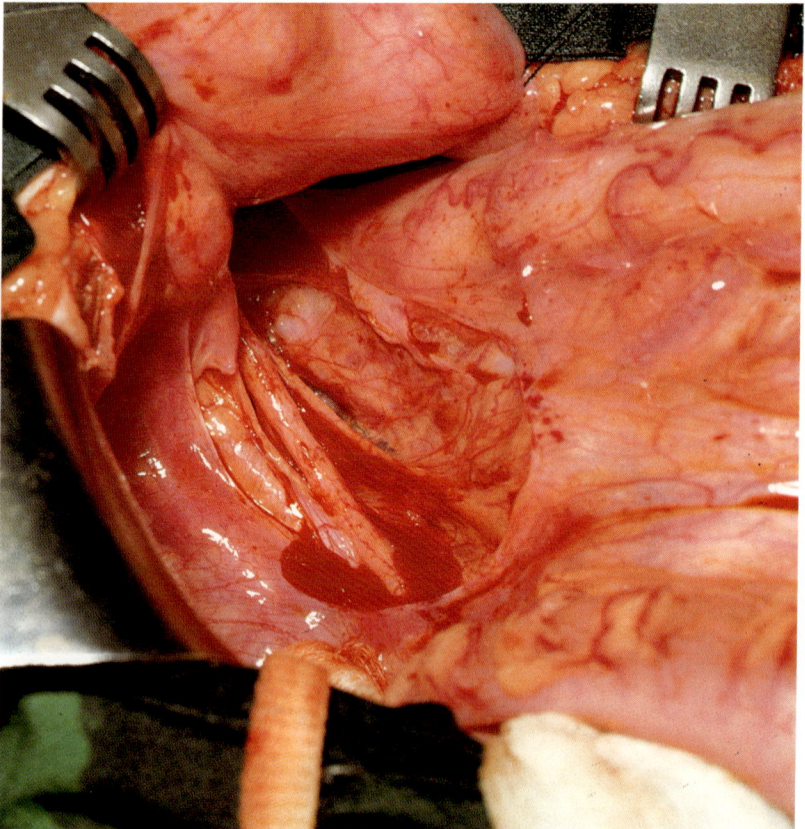

**15** View down into the pelvis achieved by the position with sacrum allowed to fall back over the edge of the small table. This is very important for the endorectal and Swenson methods because the dissection has to go right down to the levator floor – lower than even the usual low anterior resection of adult cancer surgery.

**16** Division of the lateral congenital peritoneal fold to mobilise the sigmoid colon and visualise the ureter which may be drawn up medially into the lengthened sigmoid mesentery.

18

**17** Mobilisation achieved (note the position of the ureter).

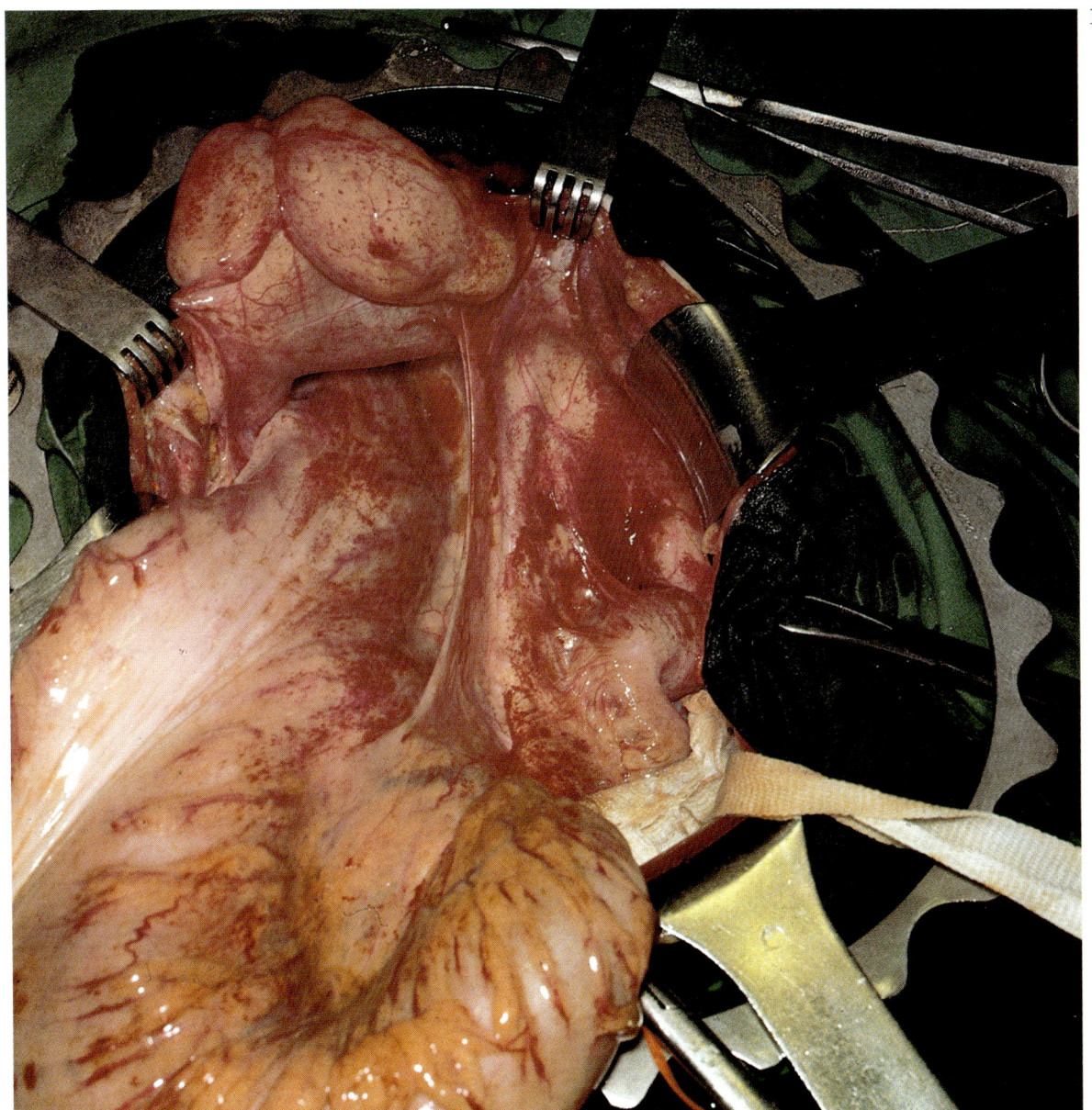

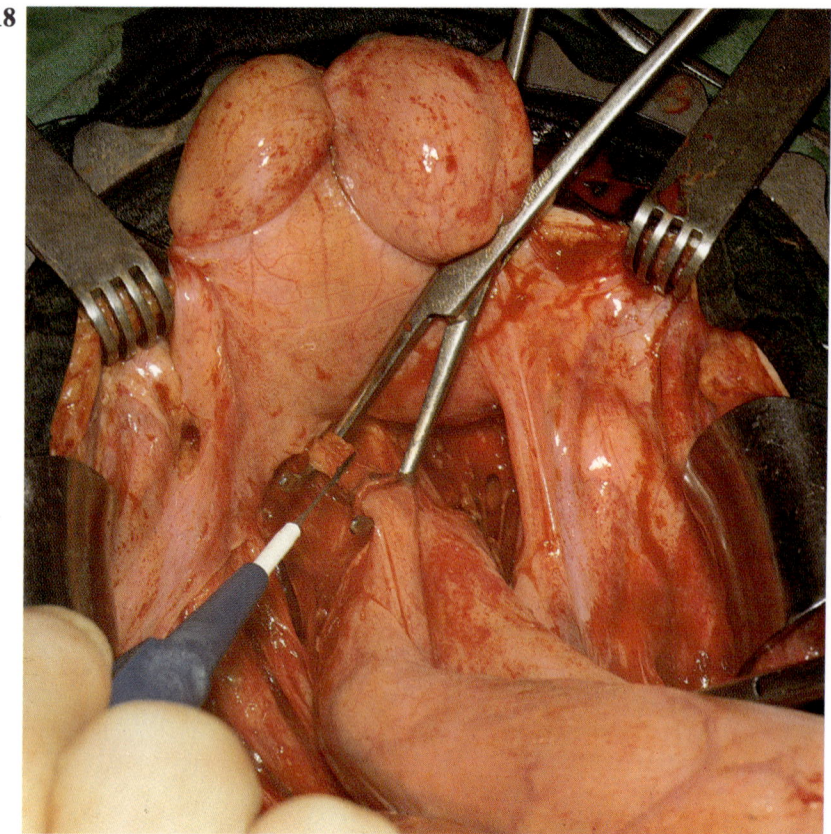

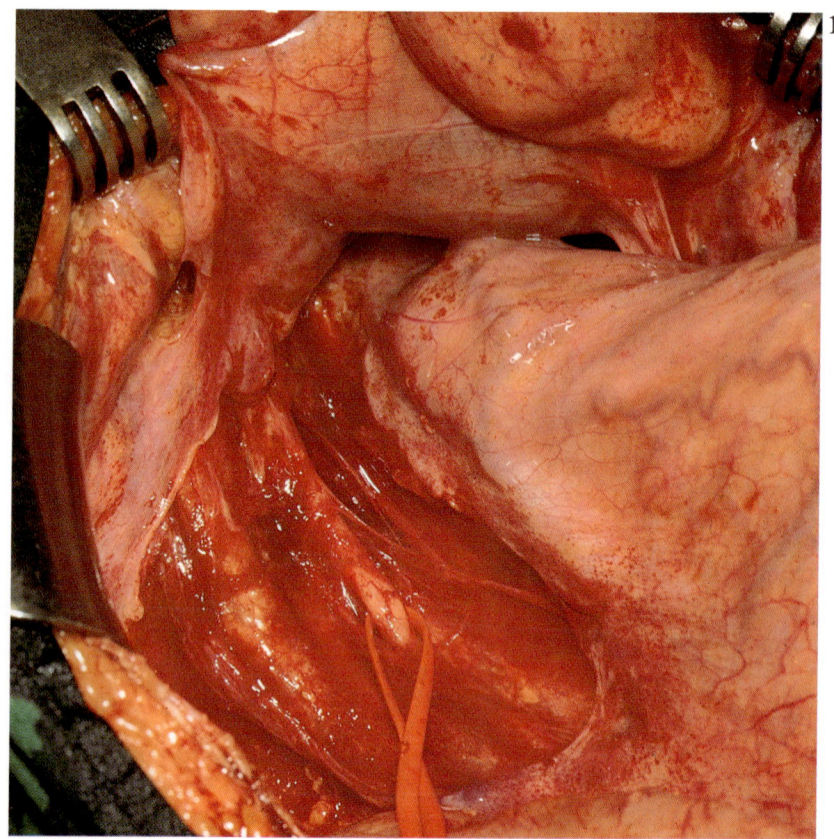

**18 and 19    Division of the peritoneum is carried around its lateral and anterior reflection from the rectum exposing the muscle coat of the rectum.** (This is the plane which must be maintained throughout the dissection in the Swenson rectosigmoidectomy operation and also in the less extensive dissection for the Duhamel.

20 A typical 'cone' of transition from enlarged normal colon through the transitional segment to the unexpanded (not necessarily narrow) aganglionic segment extending down to the anal canal.

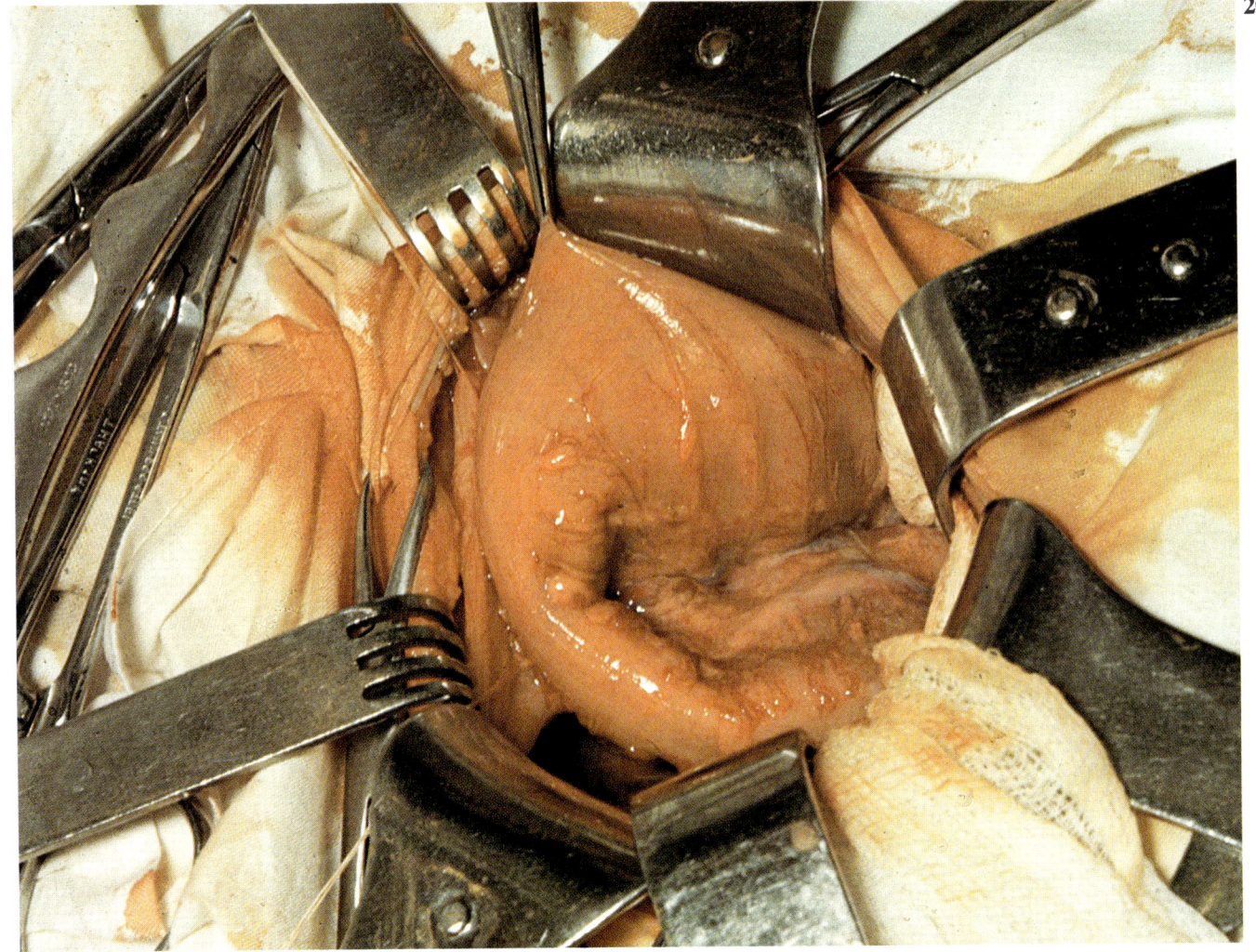

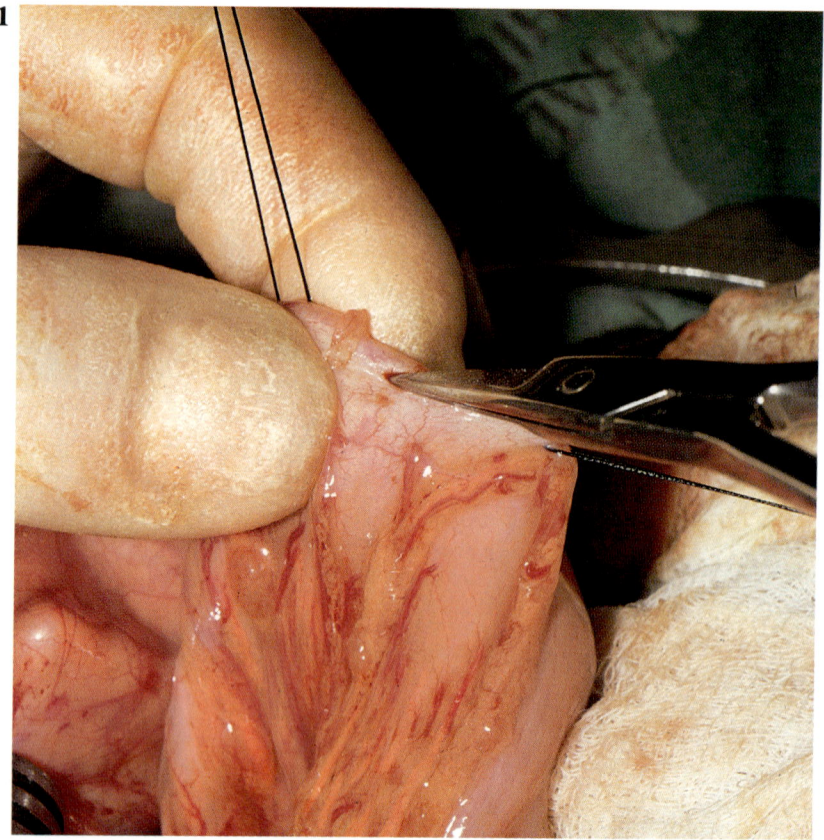

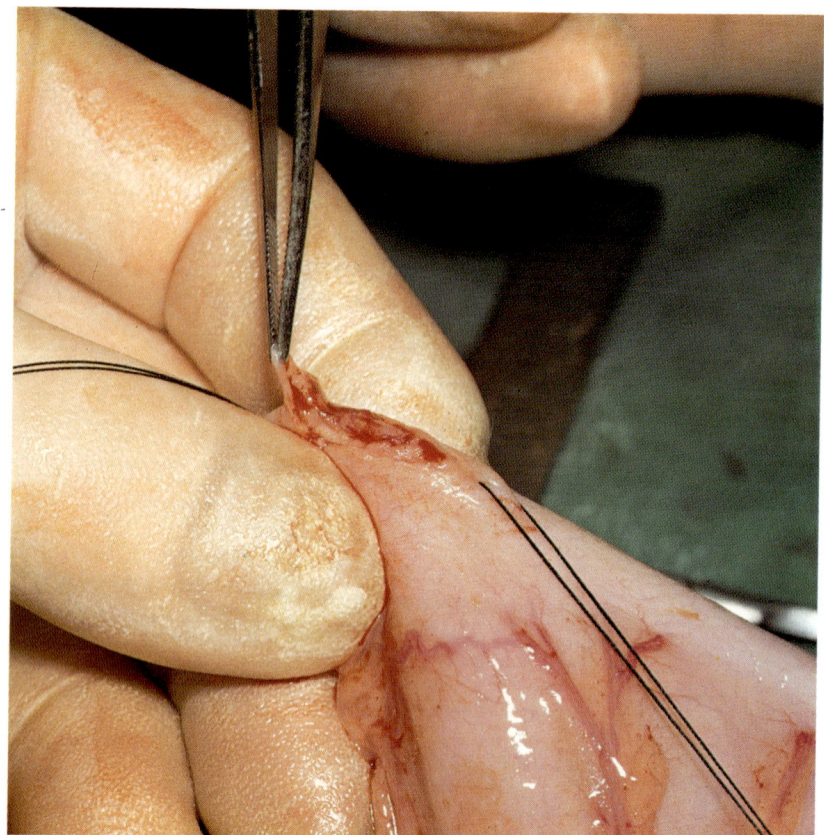

**21  Extramucosal seromuscular biopsy being taken at a suitable site above the cone to confirm that normal ganglia are present.**

When the cone is at the common level low in the sigmoid it will be convenient to remove also the maximally enlarged ganglionic colon to a level about mid-sigmoid which simplifies anastomosis and may expedite the development of a normal bowel habit after operation. It is important to remember that the bowel must reach the anus without tension. This is even lower than the level of the adult 'low anterior resection'. *Contraction of the bowel by one-third of its length during peristalsis must be allowed for.*

**22  The V-shaped biopsy ready for removal for frozen section examination.** The site will be closed with one or two stitches, one stitch being left longer as a marker.

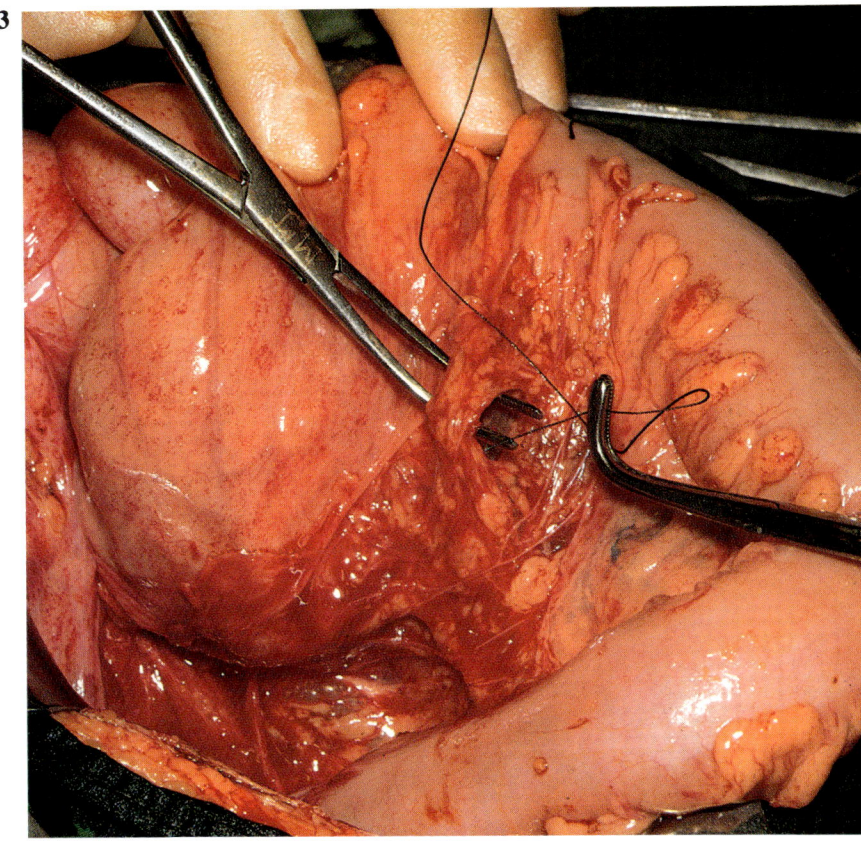

**23** Division of marginal vessel at the site selected for pullthrough.

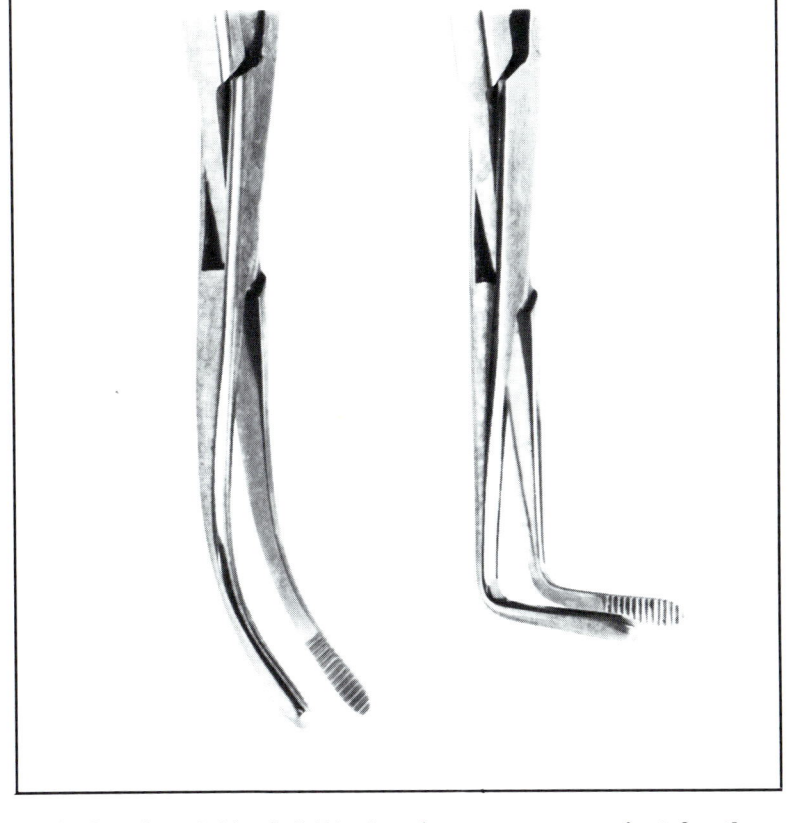

**24** **'Divulsors' and 'Angled Divulsors' are very convenient for these dissections.** Designed by Sir Denis Browne to meet and grip only at the tips to minimise the risk of catching excess tissue unintentionally around the back of vessels. Conveniently held in his 'ulnar grip'.

**25 Mesentery transilluminated to select suitable vessels on which to bring down the colon.** *The mobility of the vessels is more likely to be the limiting factor than the length of the bowel.* Mobilisation of the splenic flexure is usually helpful.

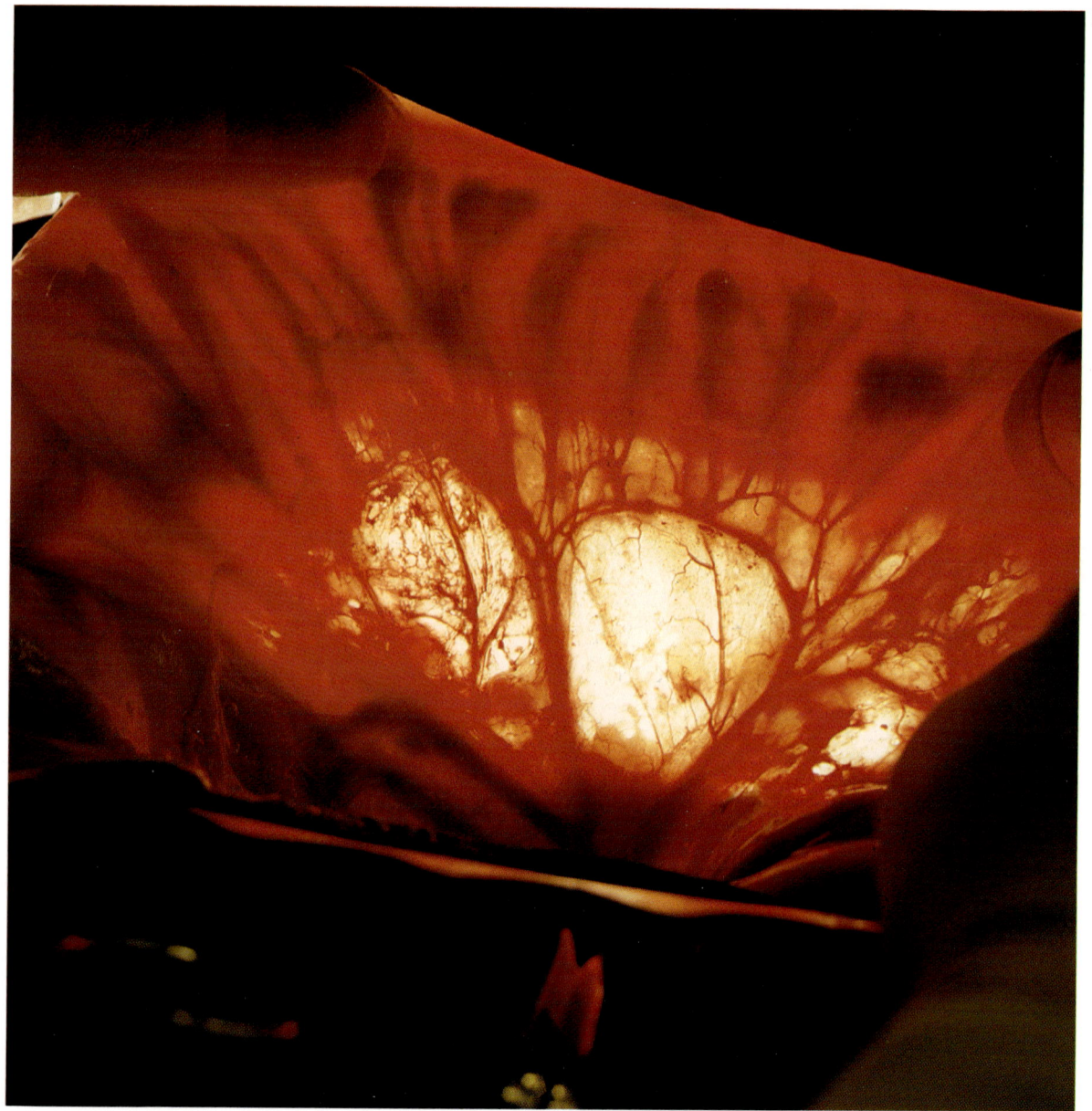

**26 Use of Denis Browne divulsors to mobilise a mesenteric vessel for division between ligatures.** (LDS stapler may be used if available.)

26

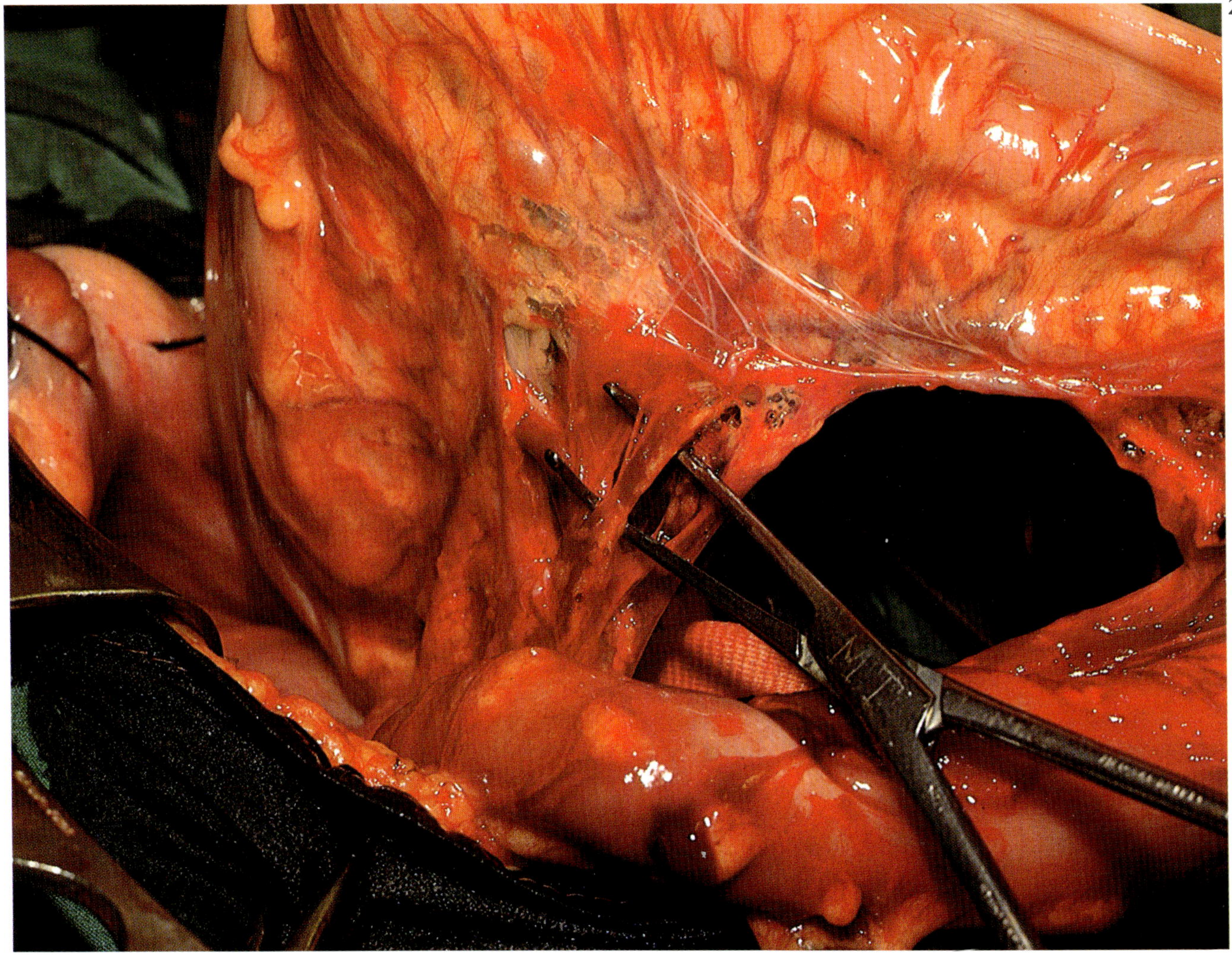

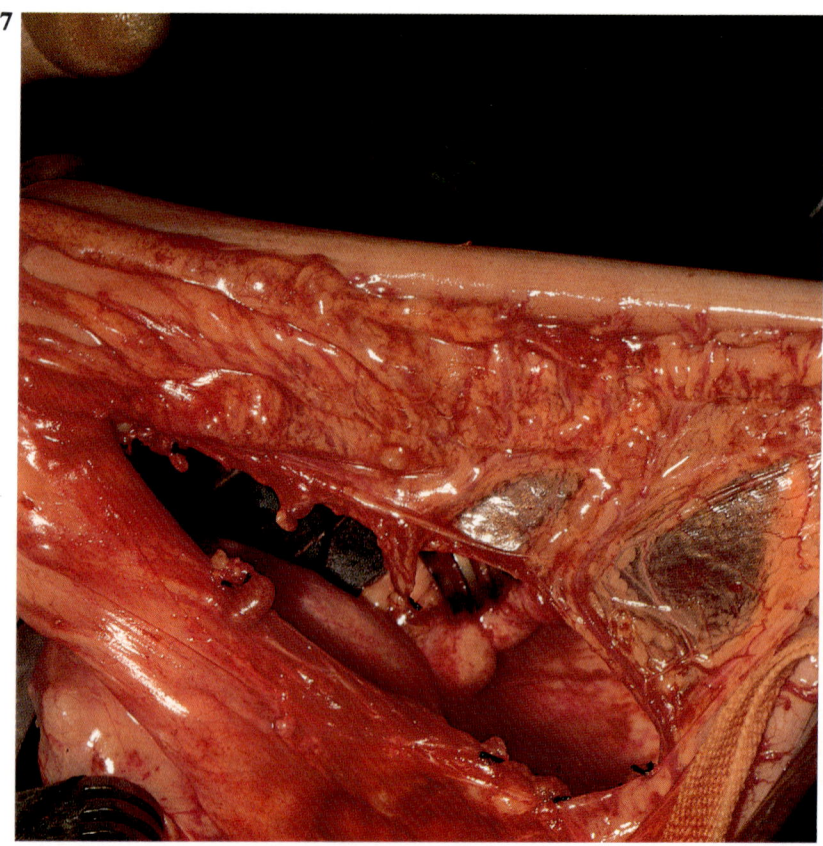

**27  Sigmoid colon mobilised and mesenteric vessels divided.**

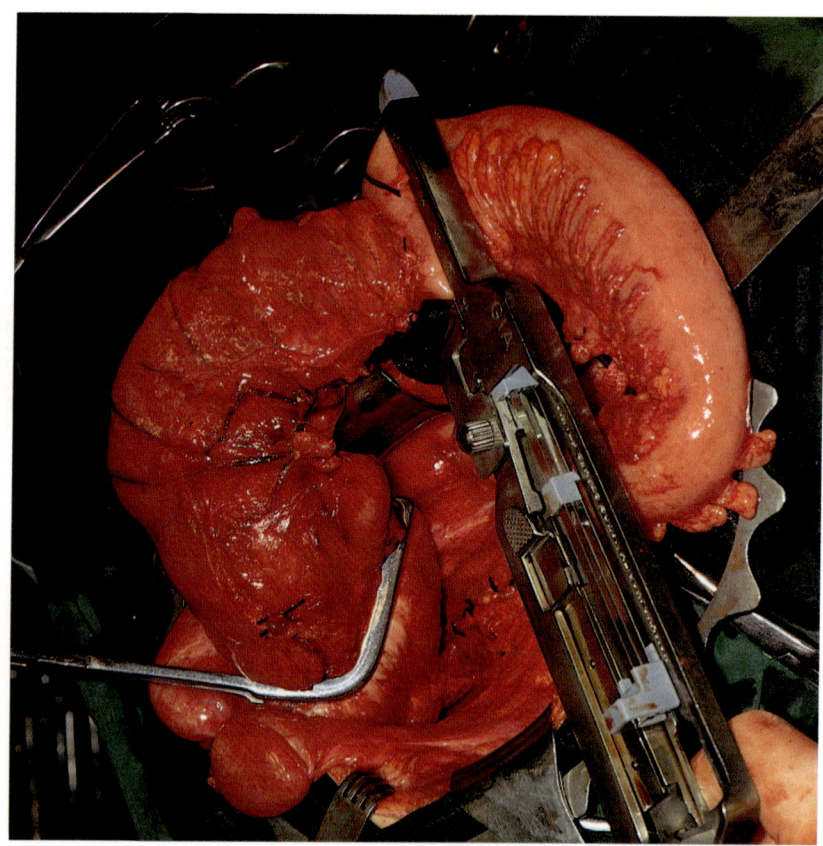

**28  Division of bowel at this site by GIA stapler.** The bowel in Hirschsprung's disease is almost always thickened sufficiently to require the adult GIA staples rather than the children's PGIA.

# Continuation according to the Duhamel technique

**29 Division of rectosigmoid 'mesentery' continues close on muscle wall till this bifurcates towards lateral ligaments of the rectum.** Division of terminal branches of vessels at the muscle wall essential to protect pelvic splanchnic innervation in this benign condition of the young (cf. the wide sweep for cancer when lymphatic removal is essential at the cost of some risk of denervation).

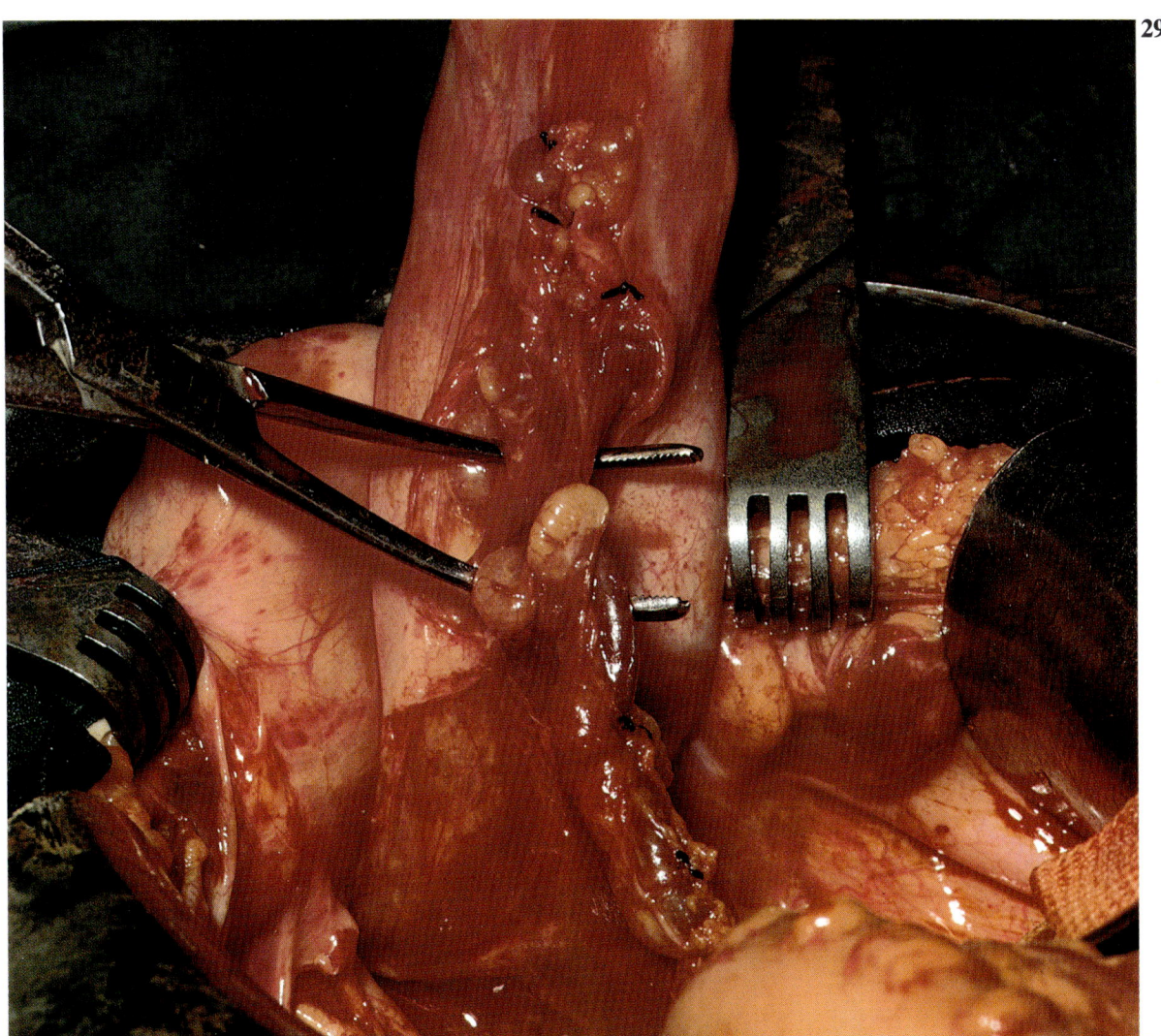

**30 A finger can be thrust down bluntly behind the rectum in the midline as far as the anus without dividing any structures.** A forceps lies in this path bearing a pledget in its tips.

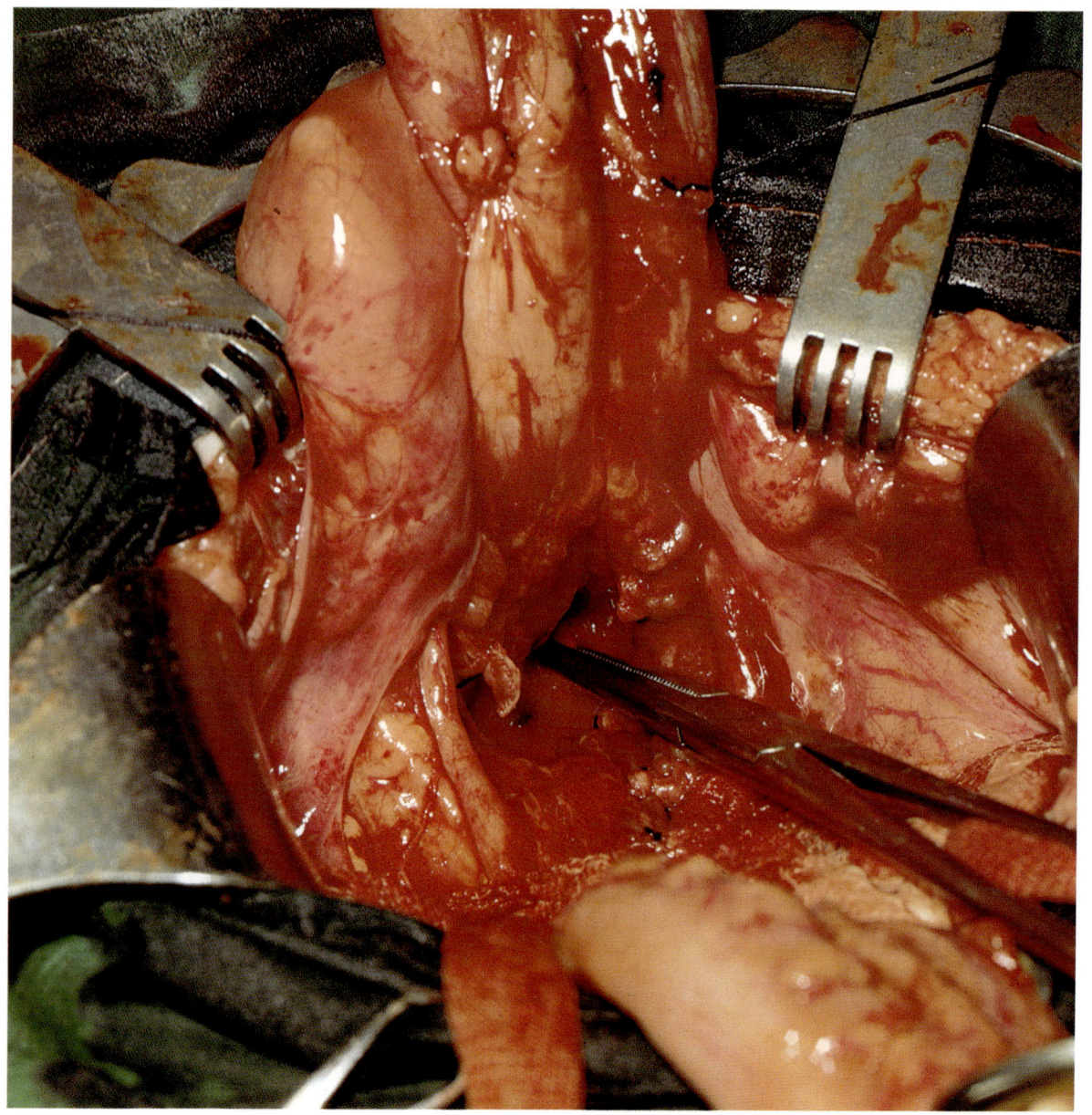

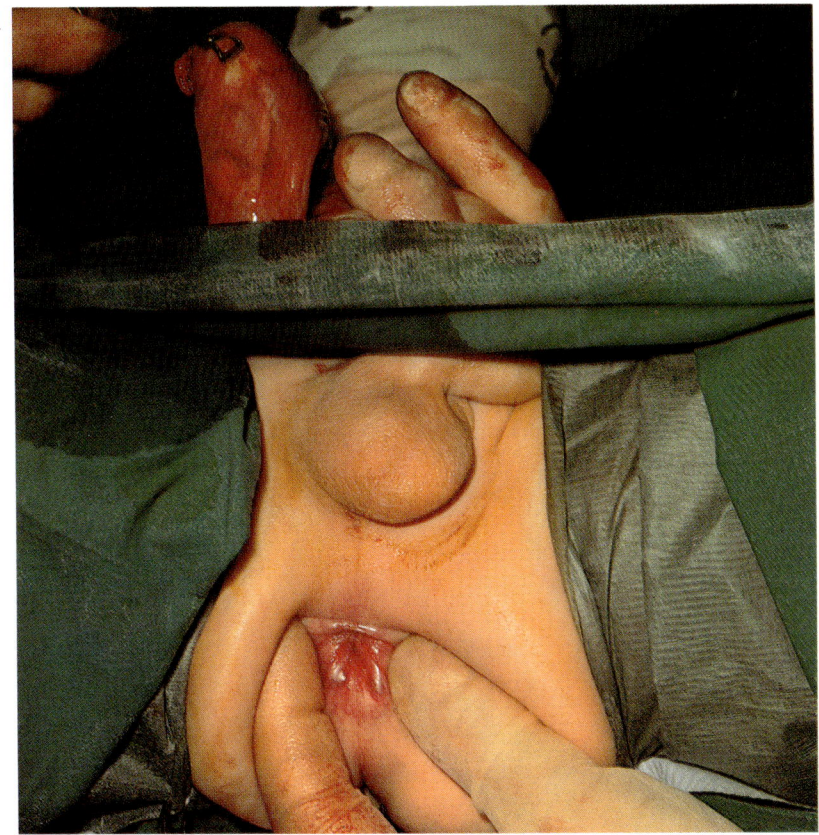

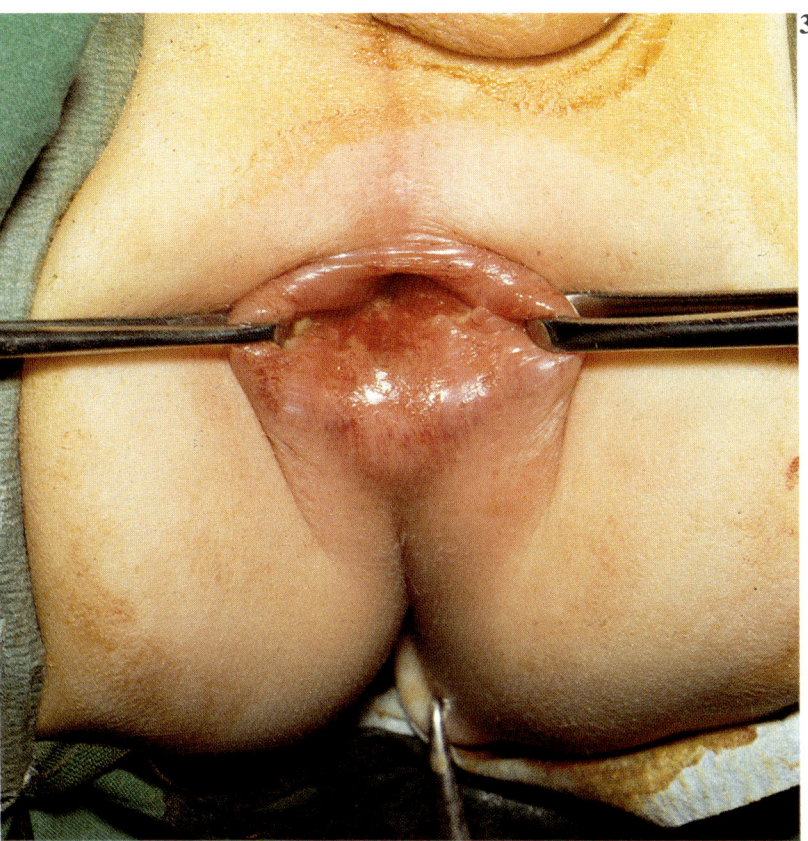

**31** **Pledget is thrusting posterior wall of anal canal down.** It is convenient to put a second glove temporarily over that on the left hand, so that the forceps can be thrust down with the right hand while the left palpates and controls the anal region.

**32** **The posterior wall of the anal canal is rotated outwards by Allis or Babcock forceps placed to encircle the subcutaneous external sphincter** to enable incision of the posterior one third of the wall of the anal canal just proximal to the dentate line.

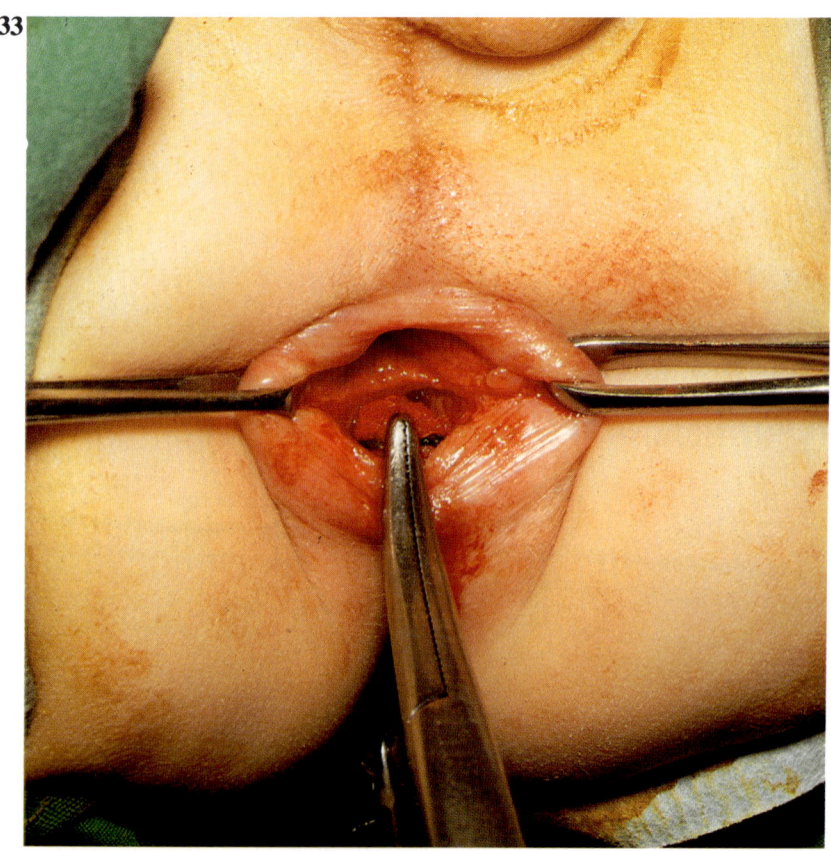

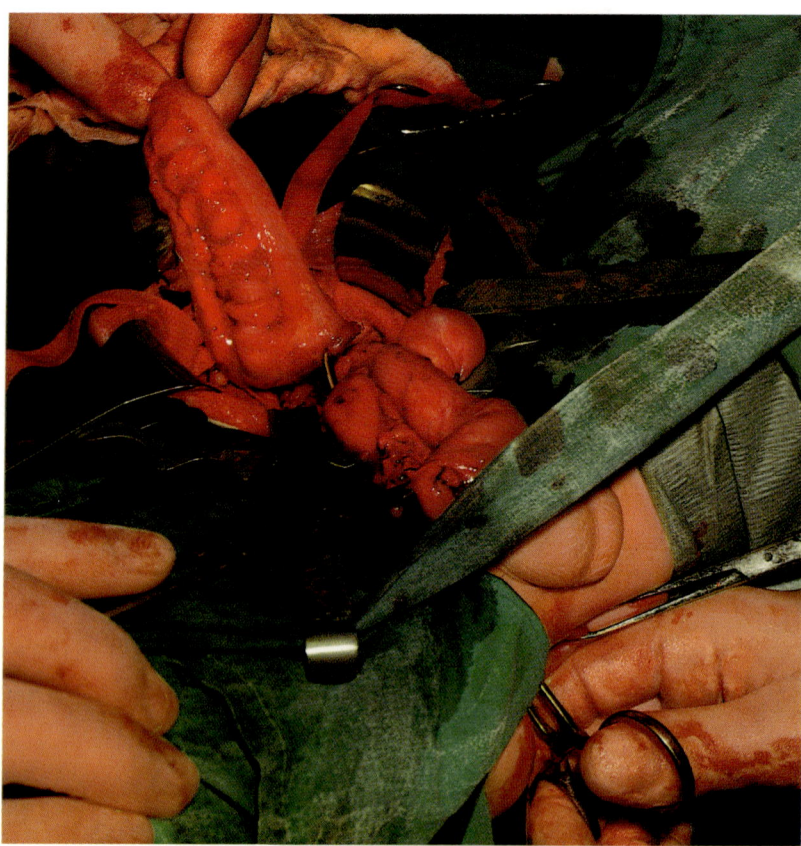

**33 and 34    Pledget presents in this incision.** Another forceps is clipped to
it (**33**) so that it can be drawn up into abdomen to catch the mobilised
colon (**34**) and draw the bowel down to the incision.

(See Introduction, page 10 for comment on extended operation for long
segments and total colonic aganglionosis.)

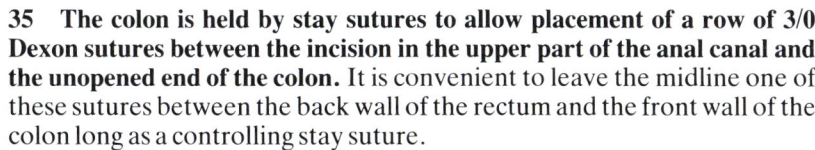

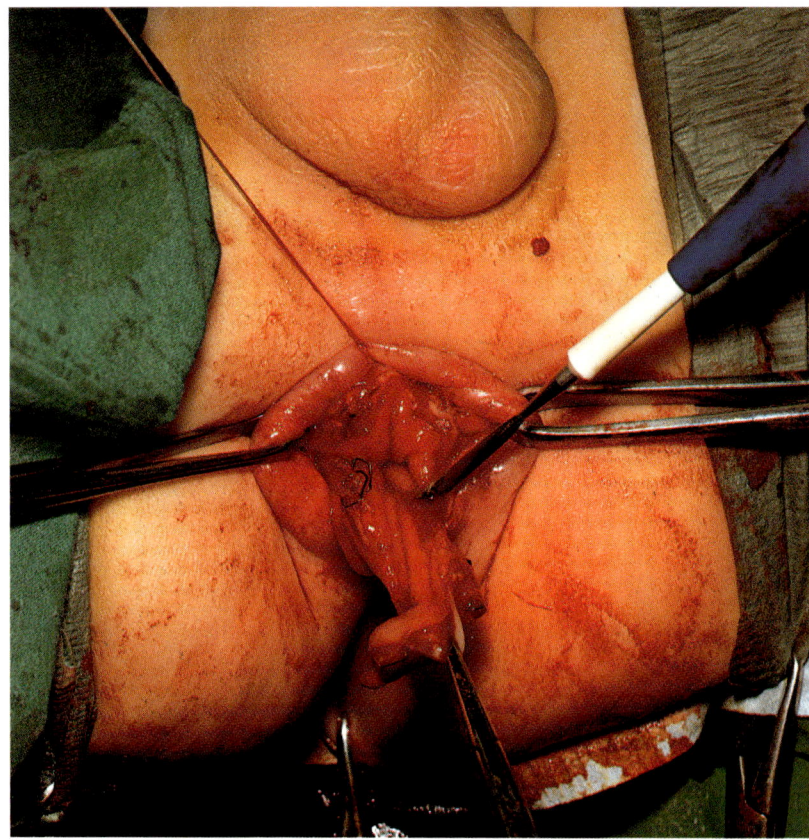

**35 The colon is held by stay sutures to allow placement of a row of 3/0 Dexon sutures between the incision in the upper part of the anal canal and the unopened end of the colon.** It is convenient to leave the midline one of these sutures between the back wall of the rectum and the front wall of the colon long as a controlling stay suture.

**36 The end of the colon is opened and trimmed after the complete ring of this layer of sutures has been placed.** There is no need for a second layer of sutures but a few may be placed for haemostasis, if required.

**37  GIA stapler placed with one limb in the rectum and one in the colon.** Adult size staples will usually be required because of the thickening of the bowel well, even in young children.

**Note** *The original stapler used here could be inserted into babies as young as 3 months of age. Unfortunately, it has been withdrawn in favour of a model with wider jaws which is unlikely to fit the anus of a baby less than 6 months of age. One therefore has the choice of delaying the operation or reverting to the entirely satisfactory, though less convenient and aesthetic, use of a clamp as described later.*

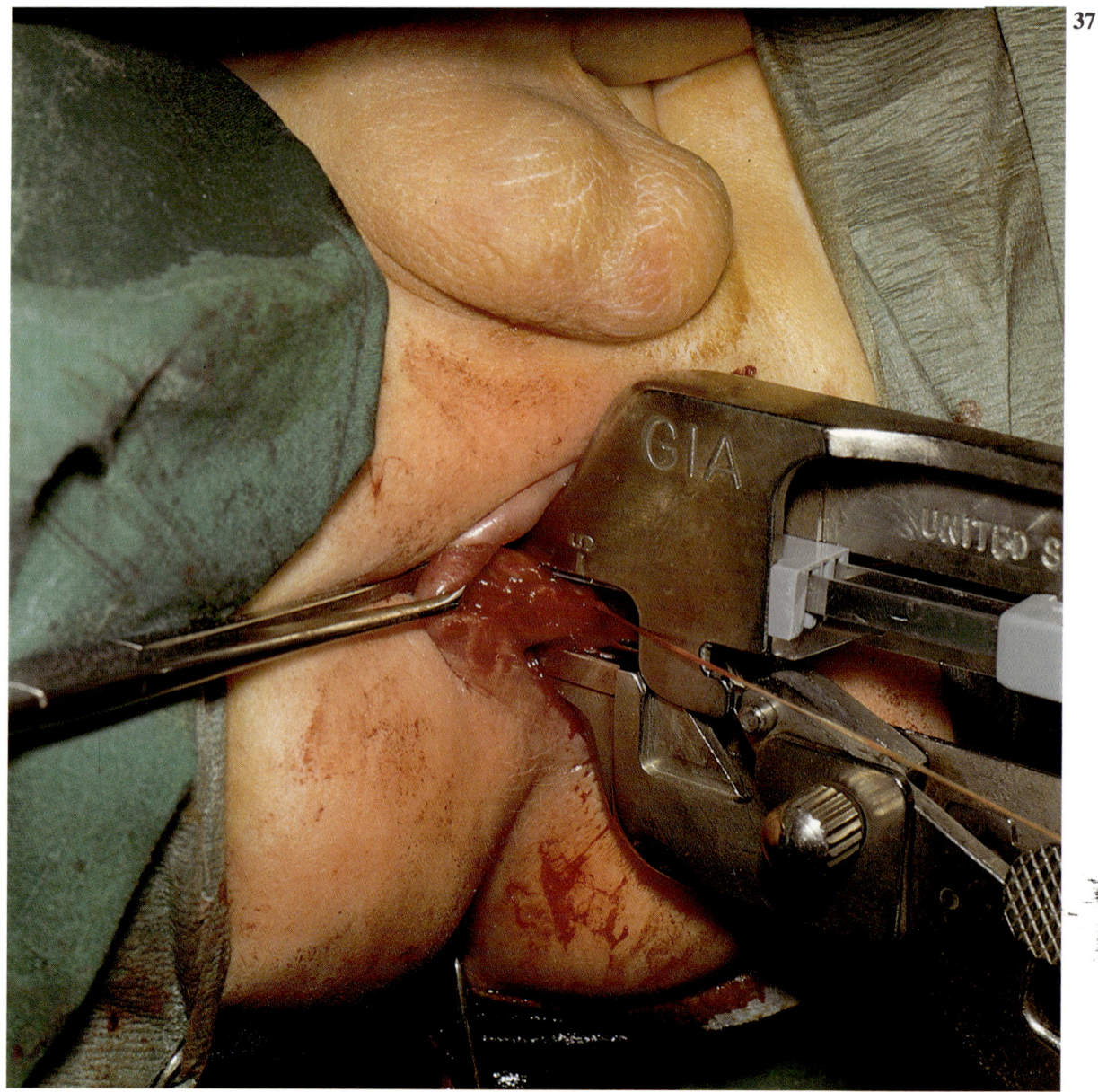

**38 The distal colon is drawn forward and down over the pubes demonstrating the upper limit of the attachment of the rectum to the pulled through colon behind it.** This is the level at which the residual segment of bowel will be removed, so as not to leave any anterior blind diverticulum of rectum. *Because such a pouch may enlarge and become the site of impacted stool stimulating overflow incontinence, it is essential to leave no undivided spur of tissue between the colon and residual rectum.*

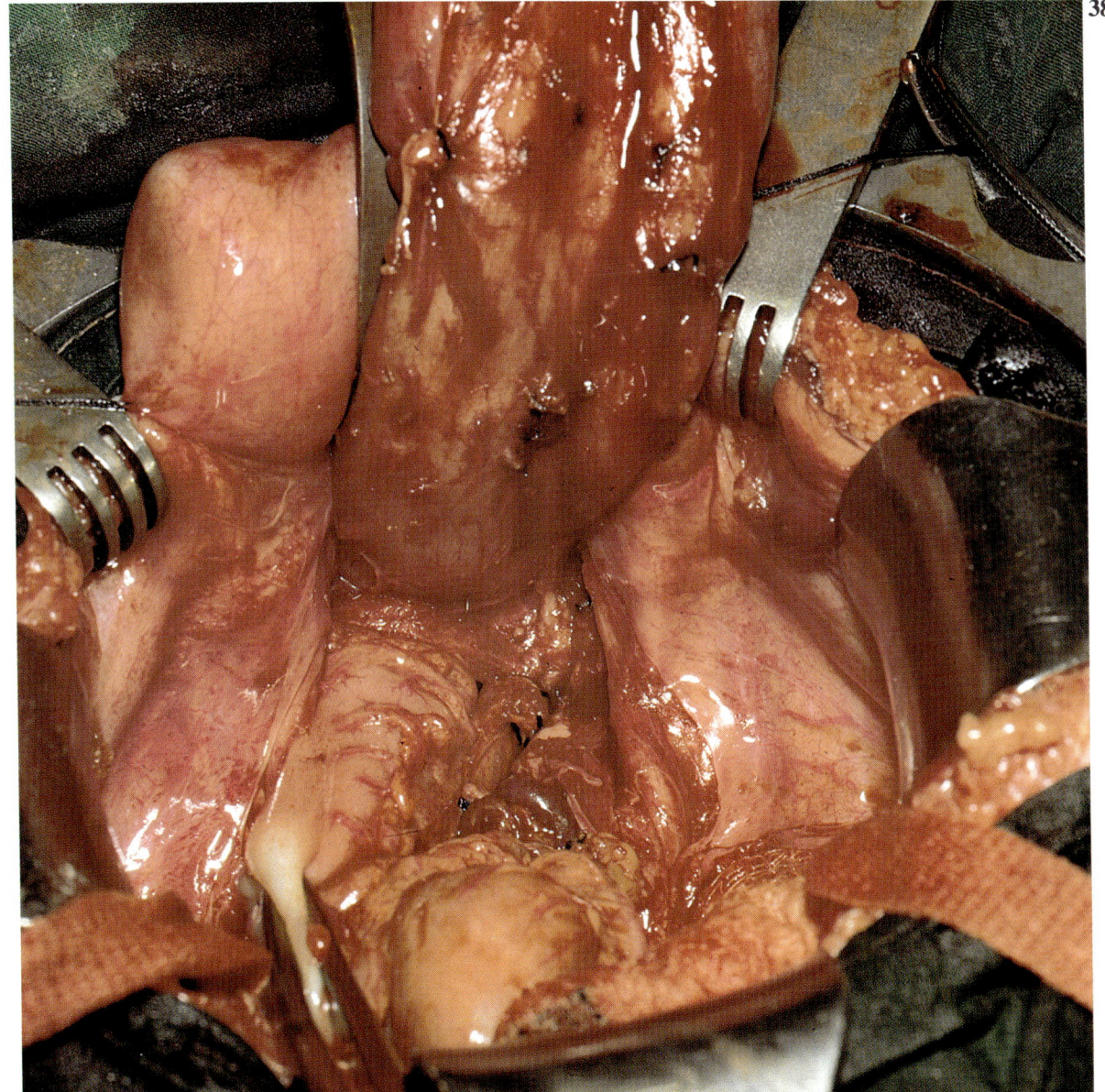

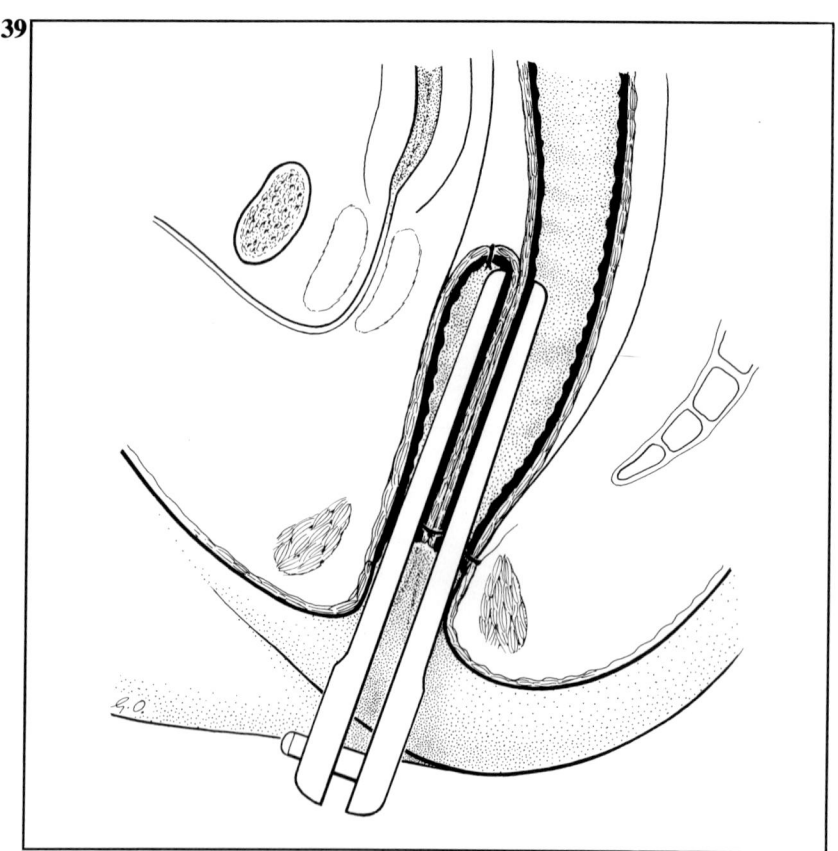

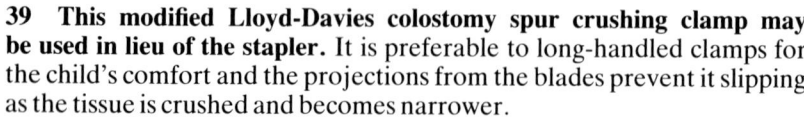

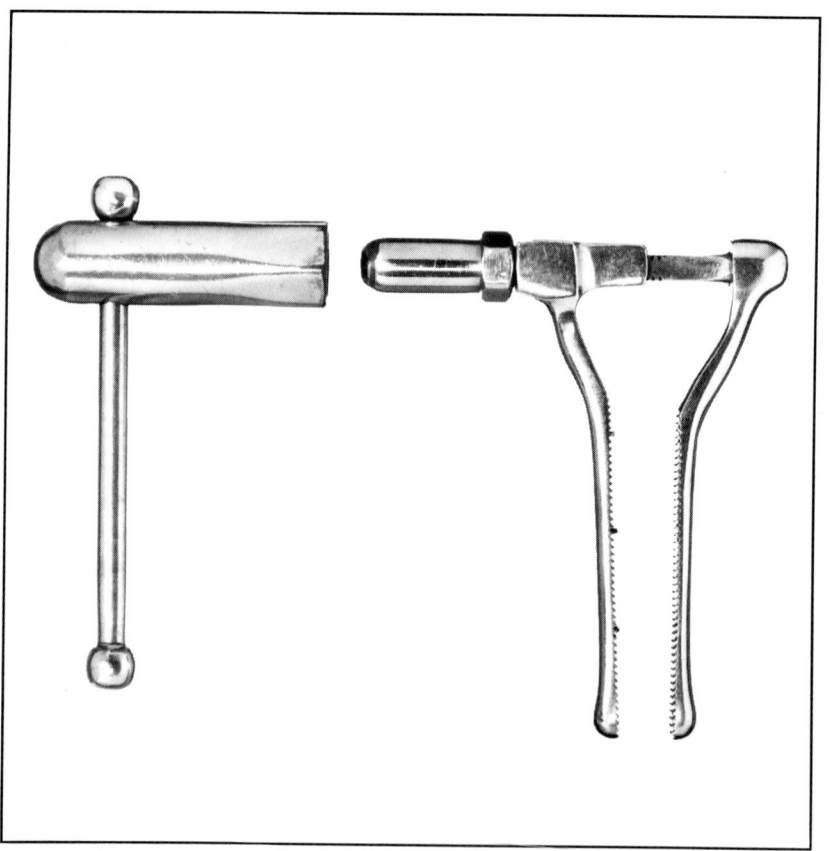

**39 This modified Lloyd-Davies colostomy spur crushing clamp may be used in lieu of the stapler.** It is preferable to long-handled clamps for the child's comfort and the projections from the blades prevent it slipping as the tissue is crushed and becomes narrower.

**40 The clamp is applied fairly firmly and is then tightened up 48 hours later. It is usually removed on the fourth or fifth postoperative day.**

There is no need to apply two clamps obliquely to excise a wedge of the adjacent walls of the bowel as was originally described by Duhamel. He also used clamps long enough to reach to the peritoneal reflection from the rectum so that he avoided dissection in the pelvis completely and had a serous coat to cover the closure of the rectal stump. *These potential safety factors are lost in the stapler modification described, but seem unimportant at least if all the operations are covered by a colostomy as the author prefers.*

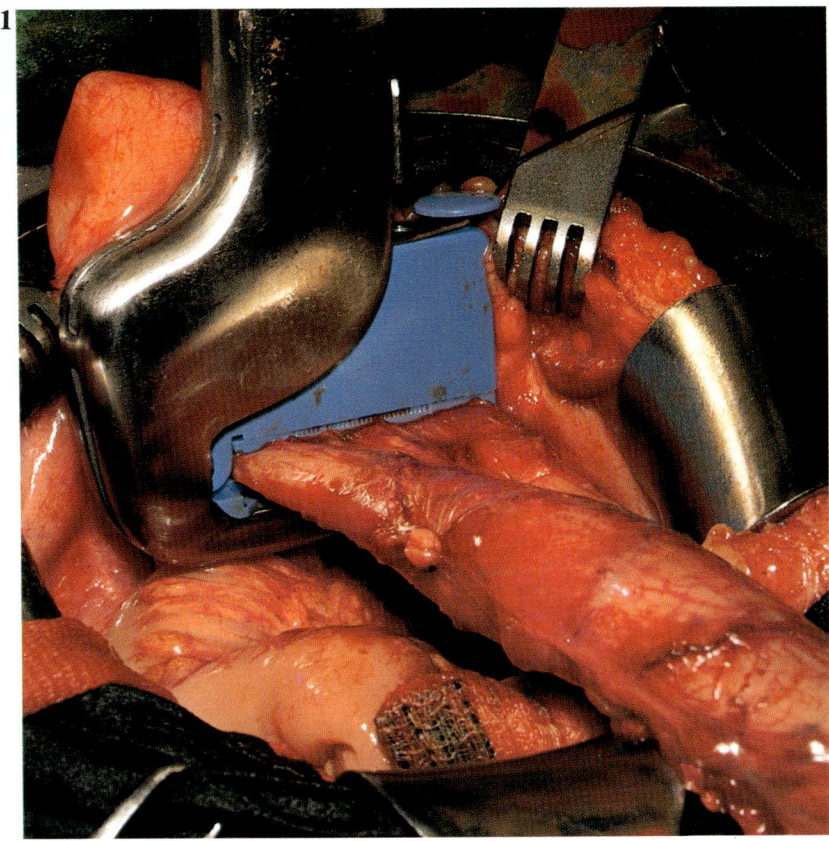

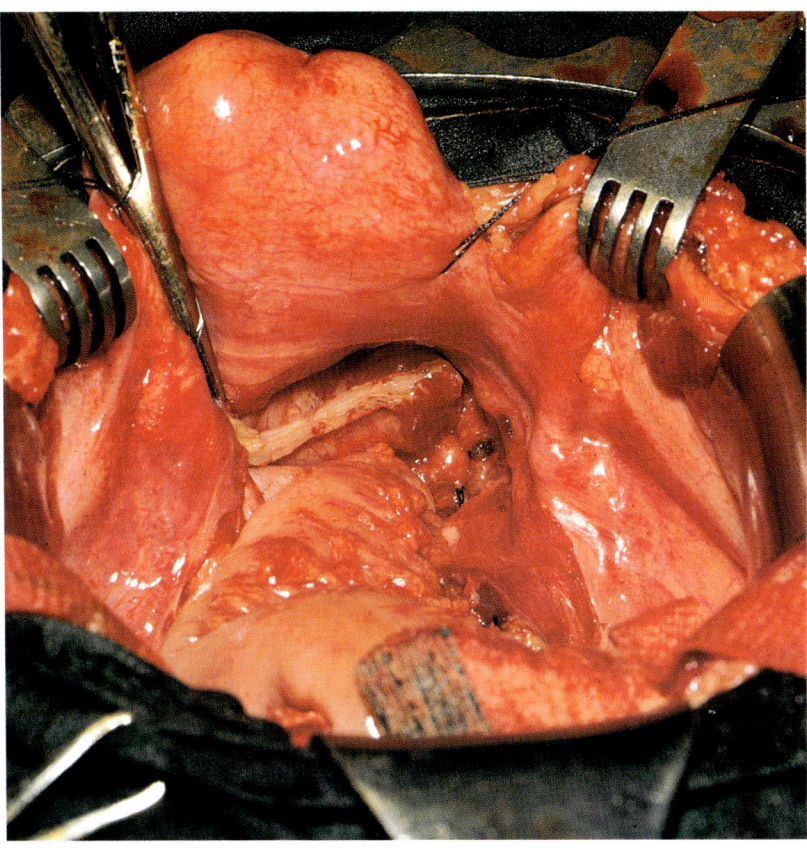

**41 and 42   The TA Stapler is used to divide and discard the intervening segment of bowel which lay between the retained distal part of the rectum and the pulled through proximal colon.** It is my custom to cover the staples with a layer of interrupted Dexon sutures.

**Note** It may be difficult to place this cumbersome instrument low enough to avoid a 'pouch' or anterior blind diverticulum of rectum. In such a case the bowel may be cut away and the open end oversewn with a catgut or Dexon continuous Schmieden stitch covered by a few Dexon or silk interrupted sutures (**43**: see following page).

An alternative is to make the pouch longer. This may be achieved by reintroducing the GIA stapler from above – a method I dislike because it involves further opening of the colon within the abdomen. It may be possible to draw down the edges of the stapled division of the adjacent bowel walls to re-apply the stapler from below. Alternatively, the crushing clamp which was used before the stapler was available is longer (15 cm against the 5 cm of the stapler). It avoids this problem.

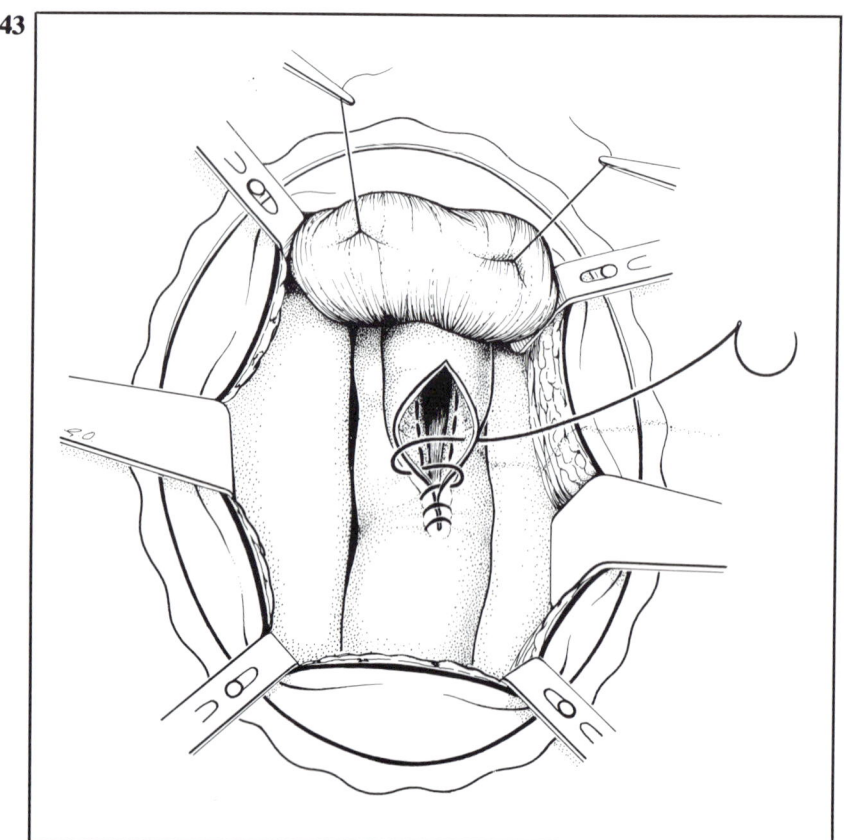

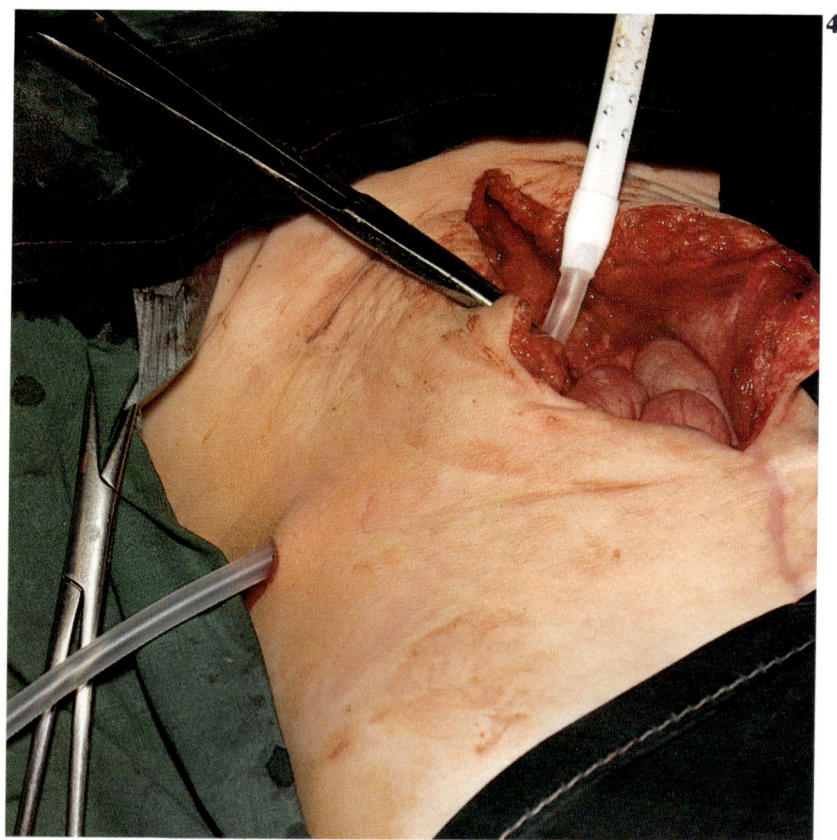

44    A stab wound is made in the left iliac fossa for a Jackson Pratt suction drain.

**45** **Drain being laid in pelvis.** Low-pressure suction is usually applied for two days; in the absence of further discharge the drain is withdrawn on the fourth postoperative day.

The wound is closed with interrupted Dexon sutures through all layers deep to skin plus subcutaneous and sub-cuticular 4 or 5/0 Dexon. The urethral catheter is removed after 24 hours.

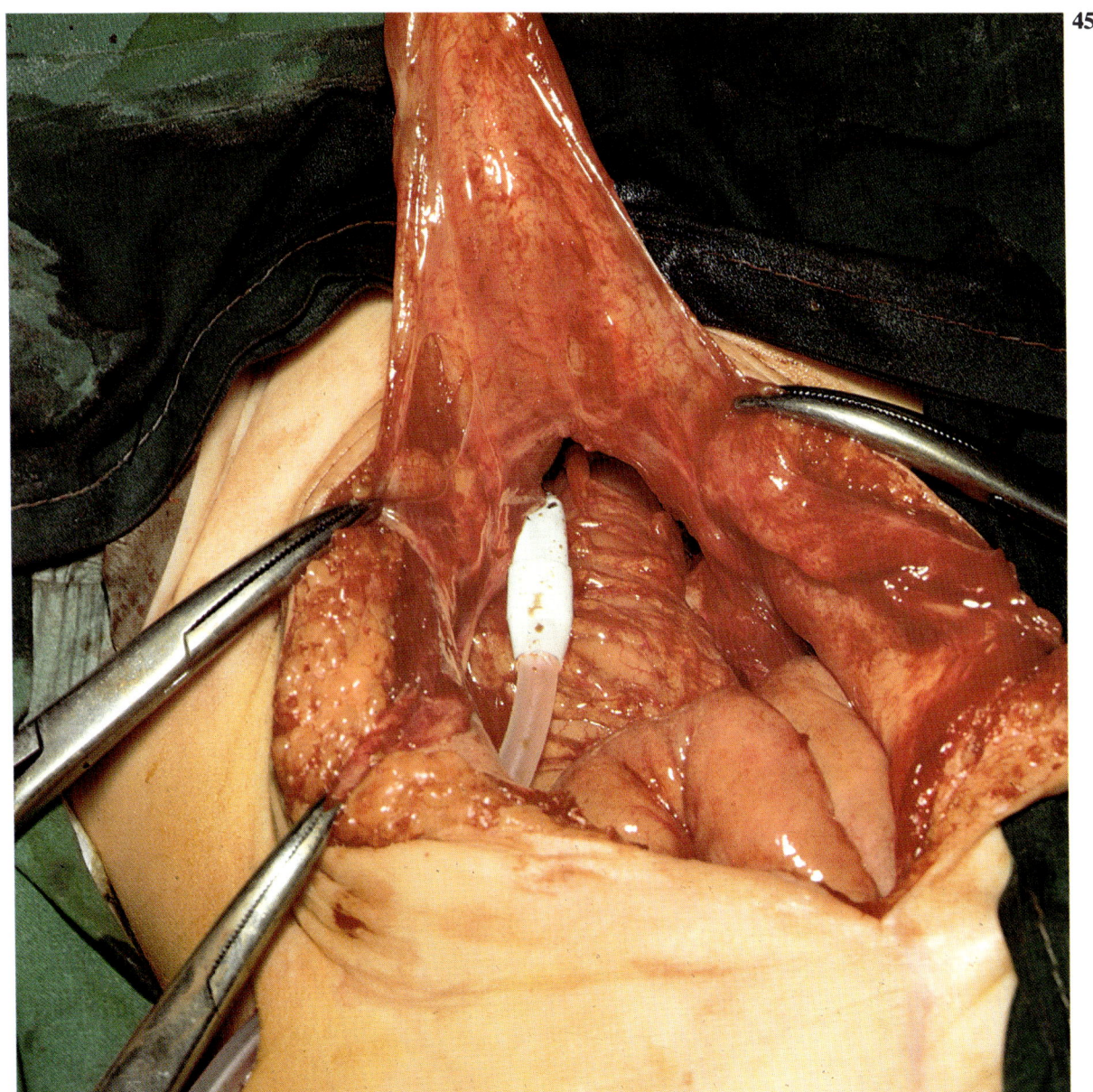

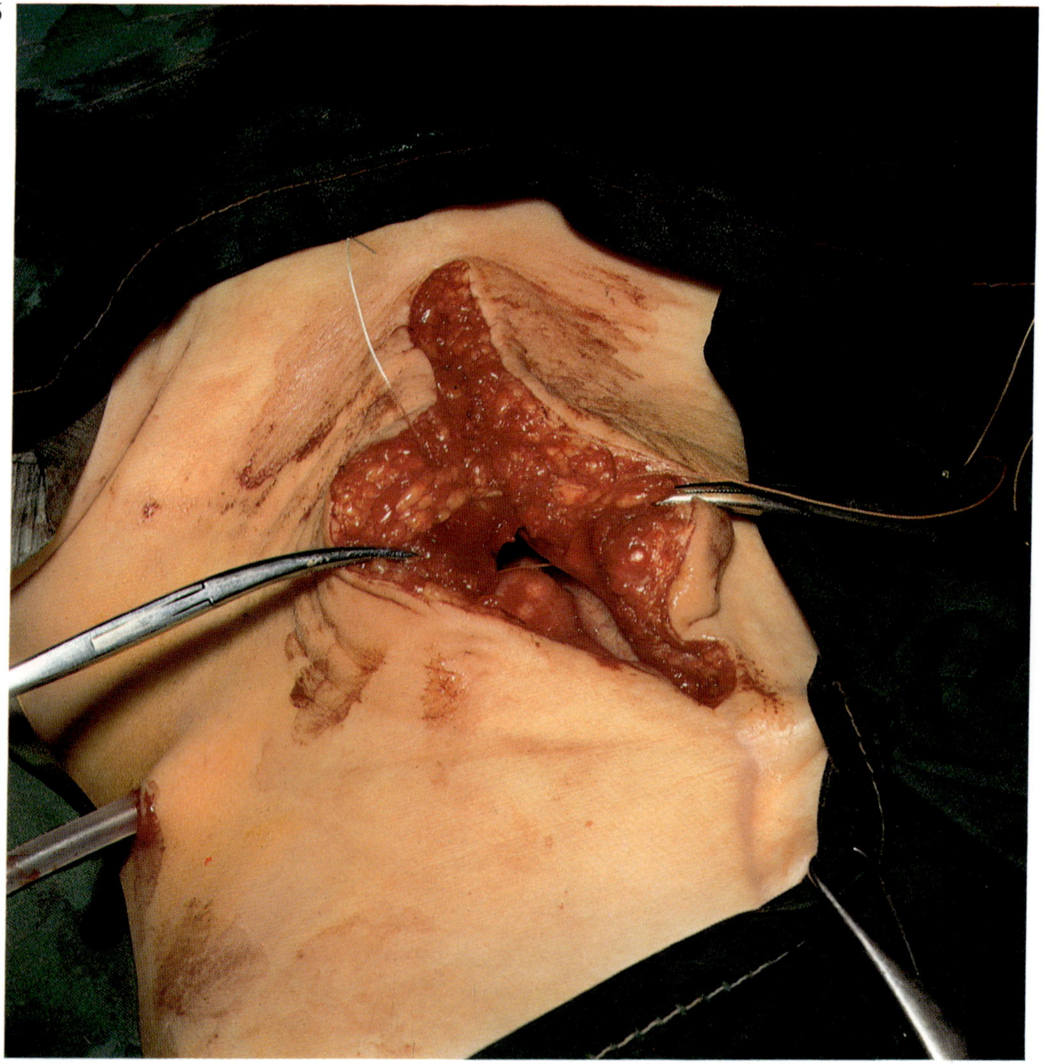

**46** The wound is closed with interrupted Dexon sutures through all layers deep to skin plus subcutaneous and subcuticular 4 or 5/0 Dexon. The urethral catheter is removed after 24 hours.

# Endorectal operation

**At this juncture there are three choices for completion:**
1 The Denda/Scott Boley or 'sutured Soave' technique which will be described next;
2 The original Soave non-suture technique;
3 The author's staged anastomosis technique. In this the mucosal stripping is facilitated by the anterior lengthwise division of the muscle coats of the rectum, and the first layer of sutures from rectal muscle to the seromuscular layers of the colon are placed as in the 'sutured Soave' operation. Then about 5 cm of colon are left protruding from the anus and may be looked on as a temporary perineal colostomy, obviating the need for a proximal colostomy. This excess is trimmed off two or three weeks after.

Techniques 2 and 3 will be illustrated after the account of the primary sutured technique.

# Continuation according to sutured endorectal technique

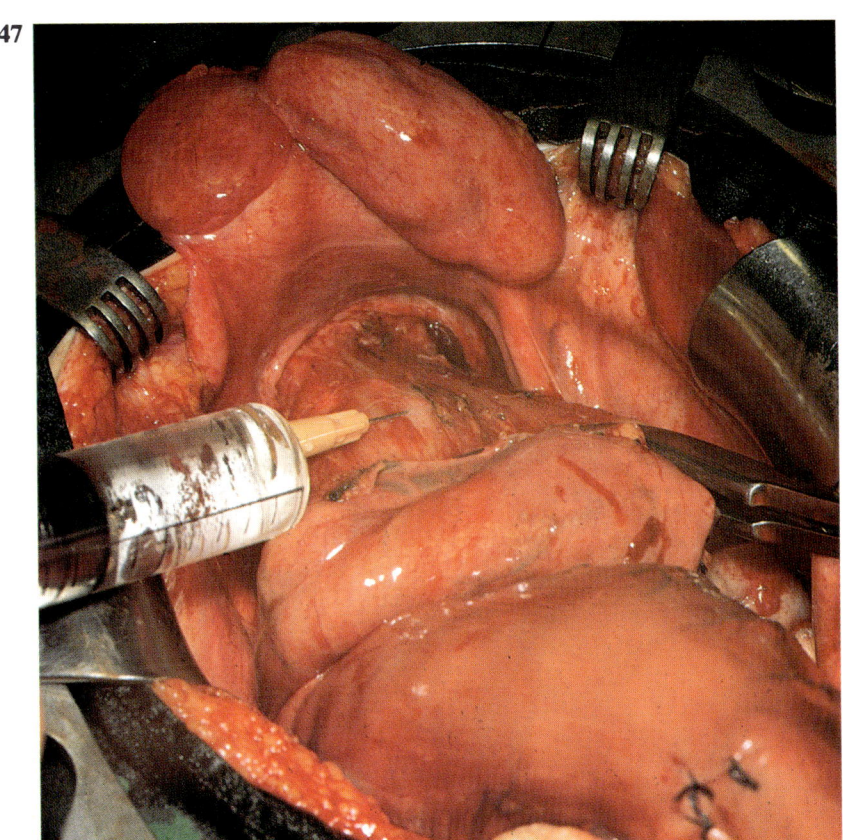

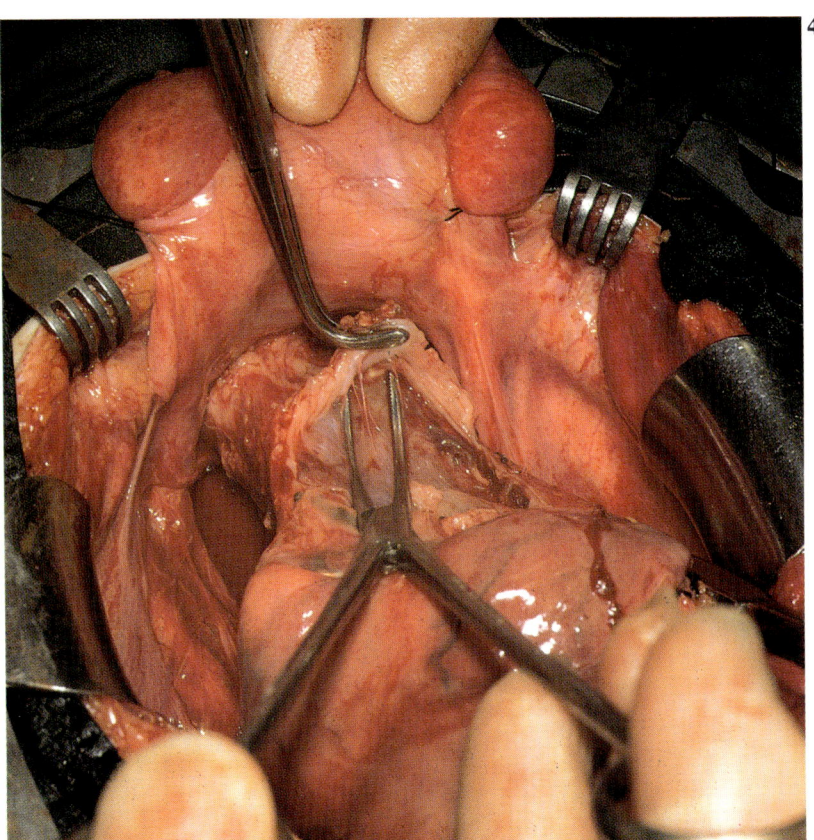

**47**    **Injection of saline into bowel wall at upper end of rectum.** 1:200,000 Adrenaline may be added.

**48**    **The rectal muscular wall is divided down to intact mucosa.**

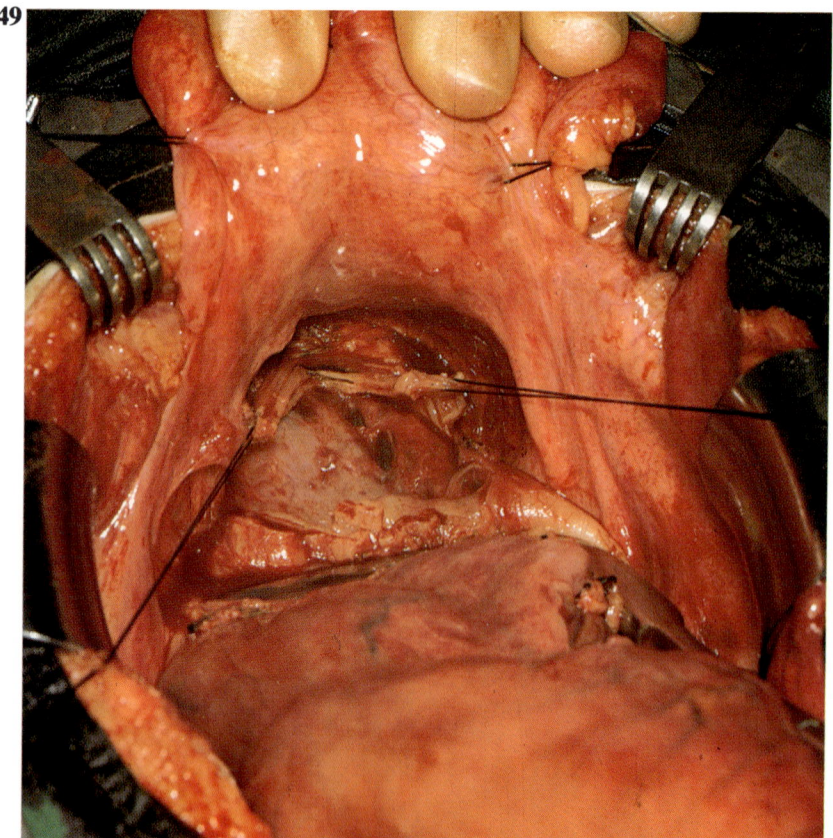

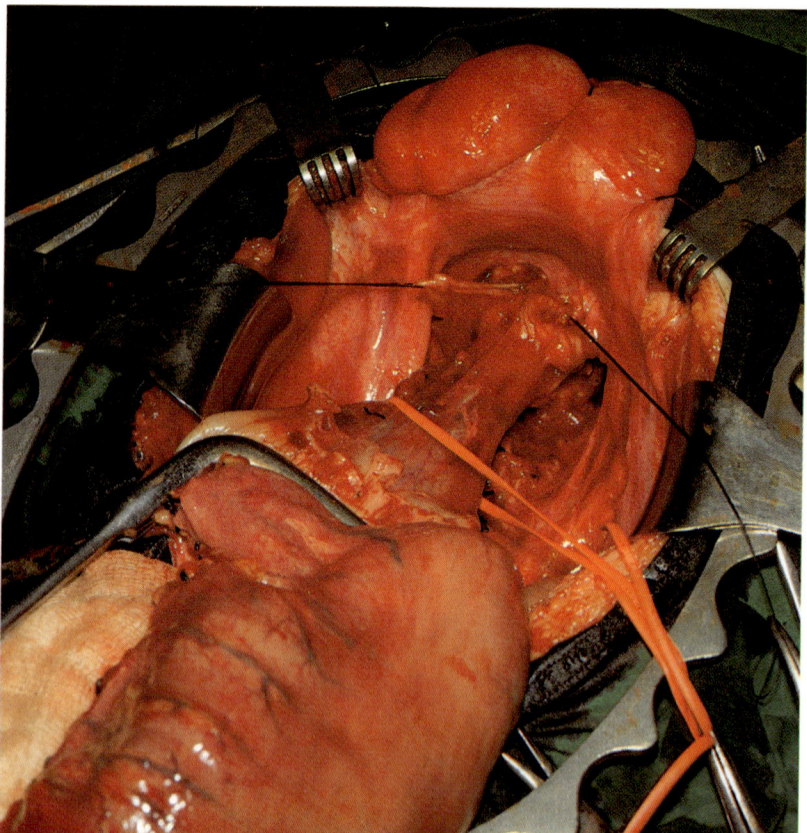

**49   A midline anterior incision down the rectal muscle coats makes the separation easier to achieve.** This separation should extend down to the anal canal and is all done from the abdomen. The level reached can be confirmed by placing a second glove over that on the left hand and inserting the finger into the anus while palpating with the right hand from above. The extra glove is then removed. (I believe this to be preferable to ordinary glove changing which carries some risk of exposing sweaty cuffs and so on.)

**50   The muscular coat is peeled back from intact mucosa and submucosa by blunt ended forceps such as DB divulsors or de Bakey forceps. Remember that fine-pointed delicate forceps will tear holes easily.** Occasional scissor snips may be necessary but separation is remarkably bloodless provided one remains in the correct submucosal plane. The inevitable ooze stops spontaneously and only an occasional touch of diathermy is likely to be needed for haemostasis.

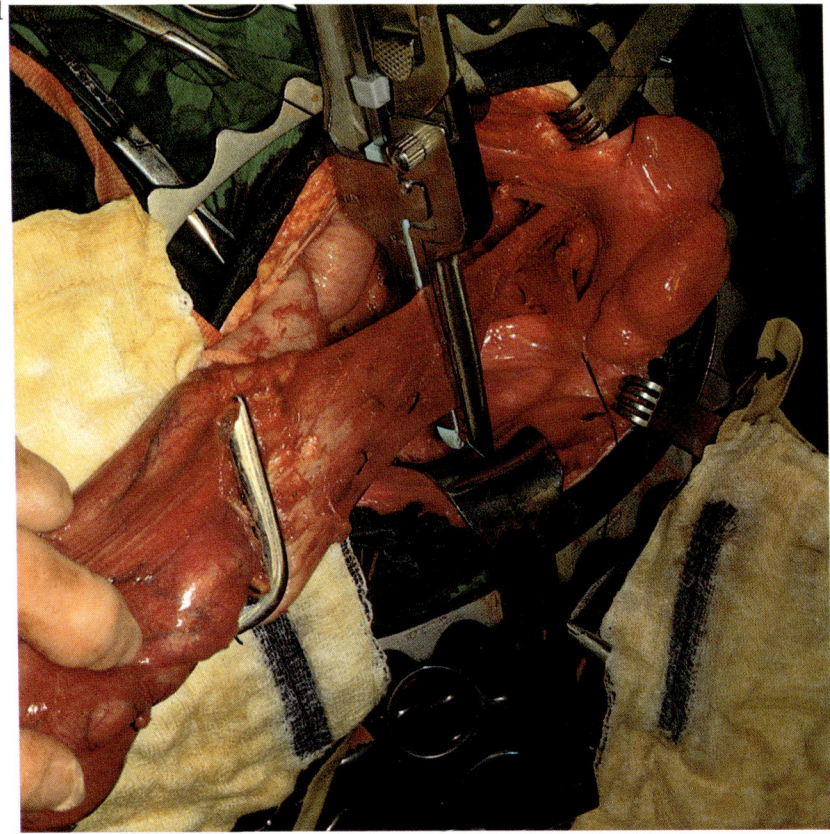

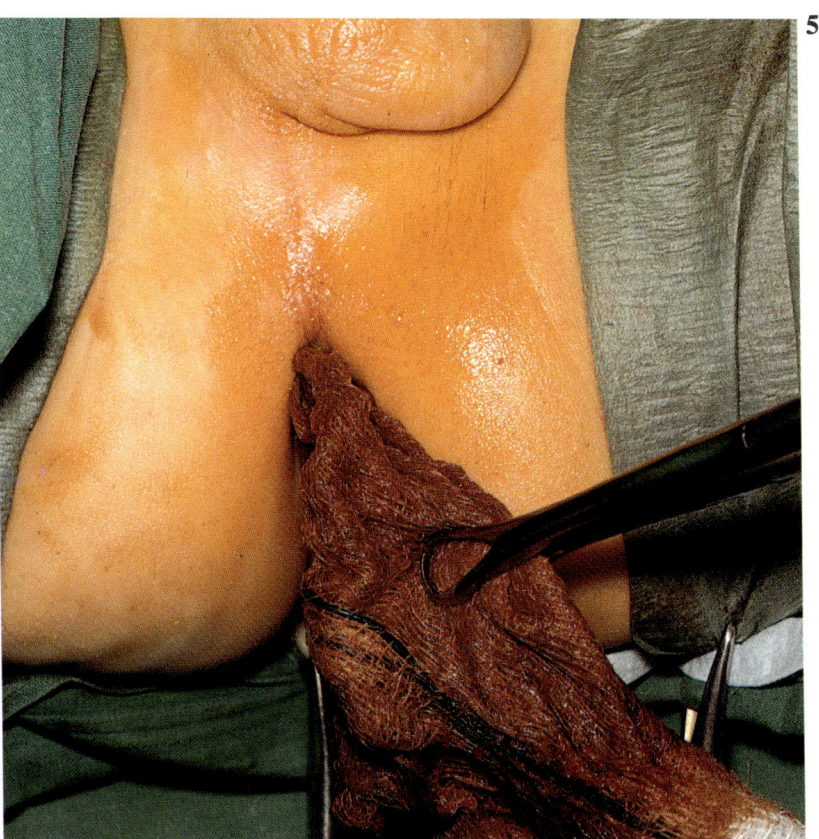

**51  Division of the mucosal tube at its upper end.** The GIA stapler is convenient but of course a running suture is an entirely satisfactory alternative.

**52  Swabbing of the interior of the rectum with povidone iodine.**

**53  Anal phase.** The mucosal tube is everted from the anus.

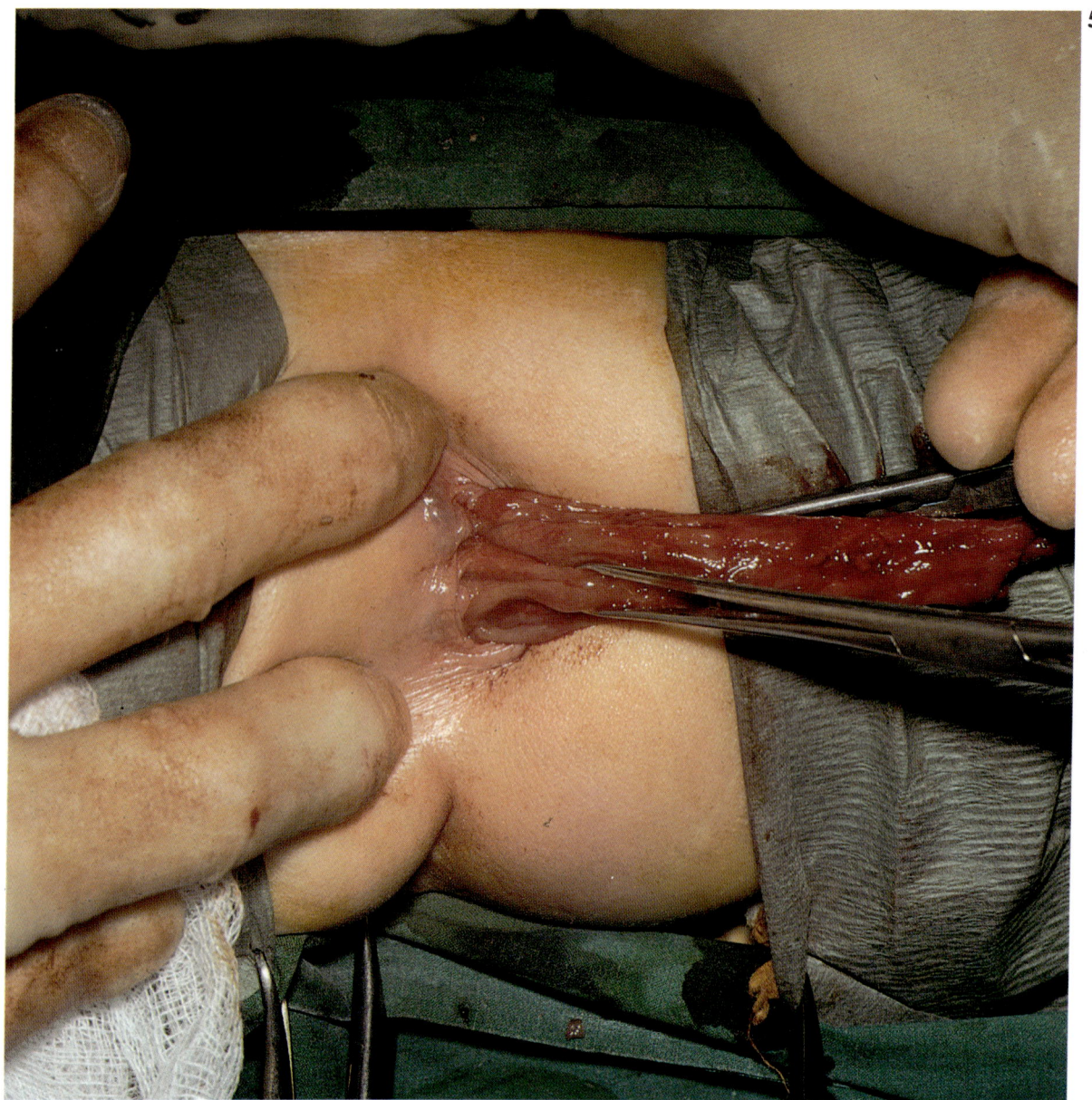

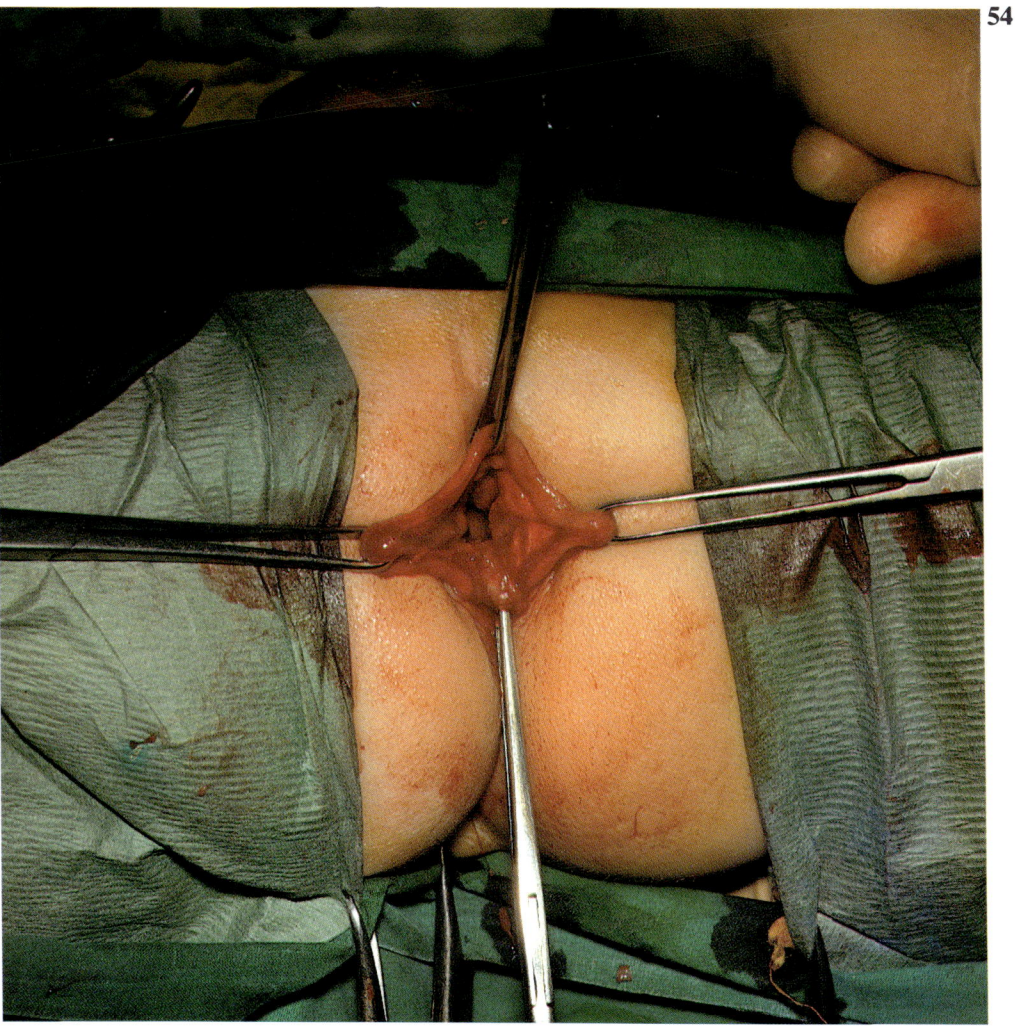

**54** The 'mucosal' tube is excised leaving a cuff of mucosa which of course also includes the submucosa. (The plane of separation is between muscle and submucosa, not between submucosa and mucosa although the peeled lining is often referred to loosely as the mucosa.)

**55 Mobilised colon drawn into anus.** A first layer of Dexon 3/0 sutures joins the seromuscular layer of the unopened colon to the muscle coat of the upper end of the anal canal. I consider this muscular suture, stressed by Denda, to be important even though sutures later placed to the colon as it enters the cuff in the abdomen should relieve tension provided that allowance is made for the shortening that occurs during peristalsis. Basically, I consider it unwise to rely only on sutures to the mucosa/submucosal layer of the upper anal canal to prevent retraction.

Such retraction can result in severe stricturing. The other potential sources of stricture are cuff abscess – which can be prevented by drainage and by leaving the anterior wall of the muscle coat open as the author does – and devascularisation of the muscle cuff by division of the superior rectal artery. Division of this artery makes the pelvic dissection less vascular in the Swenson operation in which the rectum is removed but should be avoided in other operations in which any considerable length of the upper part of the rectum is retained.

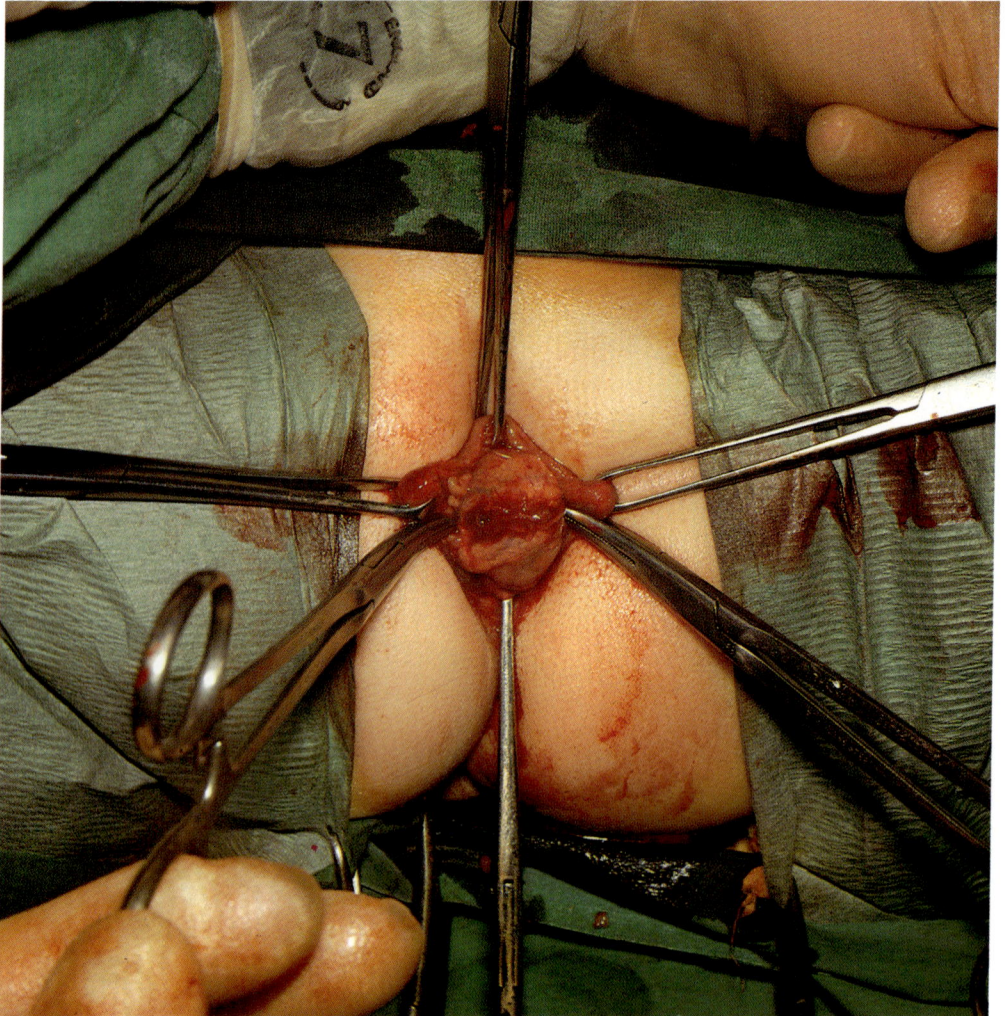

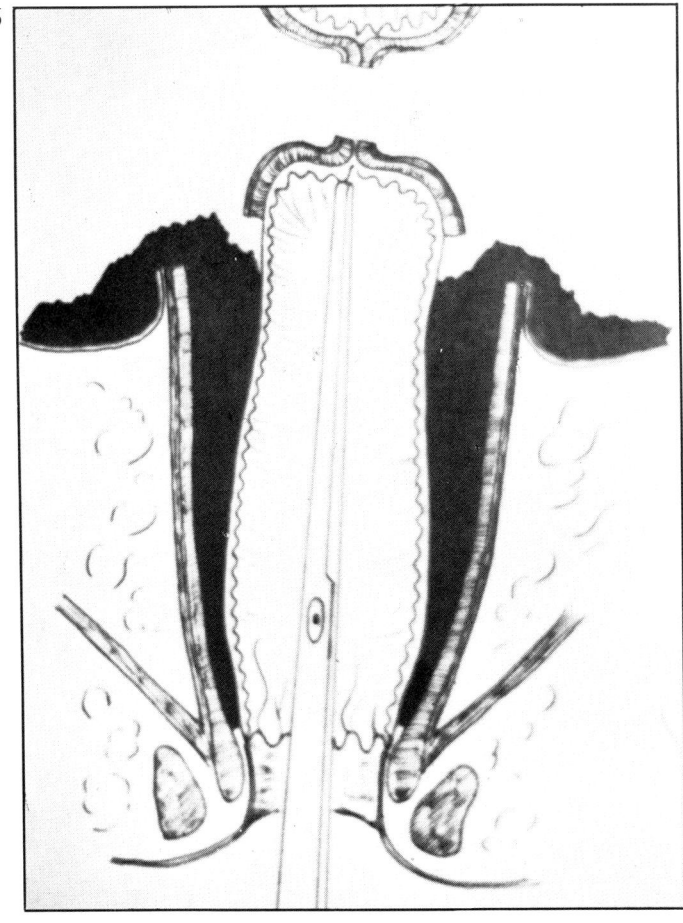

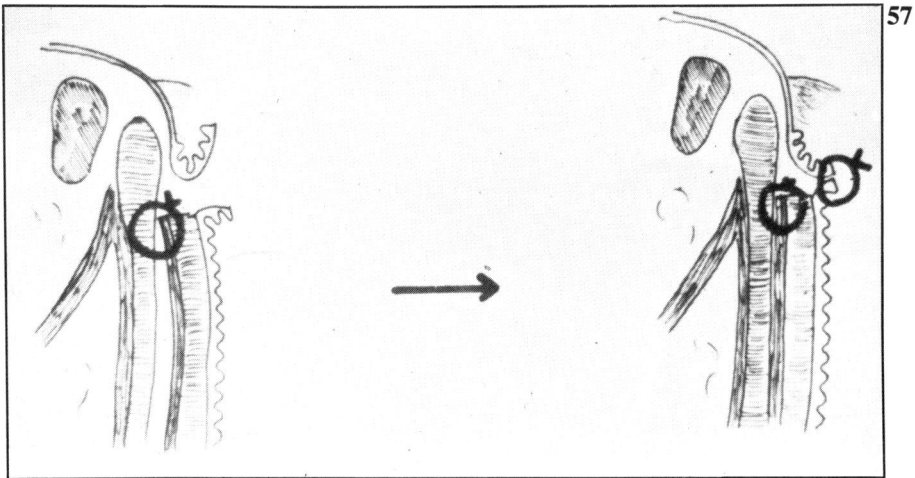

**56 and 57   After Denda** (1965, personal communication following presentation of results in 30 cases at International Paediatric Surgical Congress, Tokyo). Illustrates the muscular sutures referred to.

**58**   **The end of the pulled through colon is opened for a second layer of sutures – full thickness of colon to mucosa/submucosa at the upper end of anal canal.**
(A few sutures may be placed within the pelvis to attach the upper end of the muscle coats of the rectum to the pulled through colon to add support to the anal sutures, but these should be few to avoid the risk of pocketing of infection in the cuff.)

Closure and drainage is as described for the Duhamel operation.

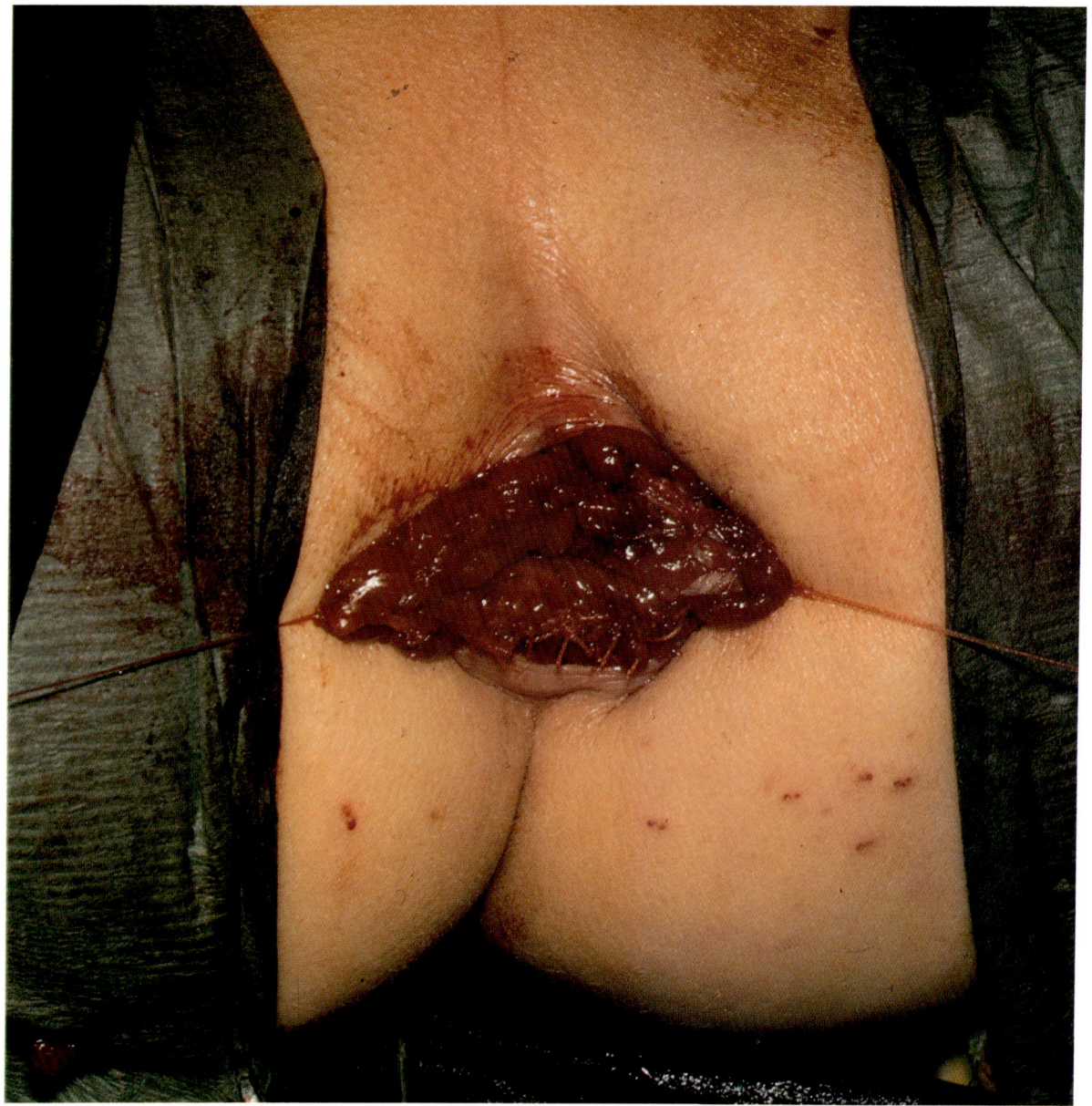

# Alternative completions of endorectal technique

**The alternatives. (a) Non-sutured, (b) The author's staged anastomosis.** Soave prefers to leave the protruding colon free to form his 'dynamic adhesions', suturing only the upper end of the cuff to the pulled through colon, leaving a soft drain inside the cuff.

In the author's modification the colon is similarly drawn down to protrude about 5 cm beyond the anus but the first layer of sutures between rectal muscle and the seromuscular layer of the colon is laid just as in the completely sutured anastomosis method already described before the end of the bowel is opened.

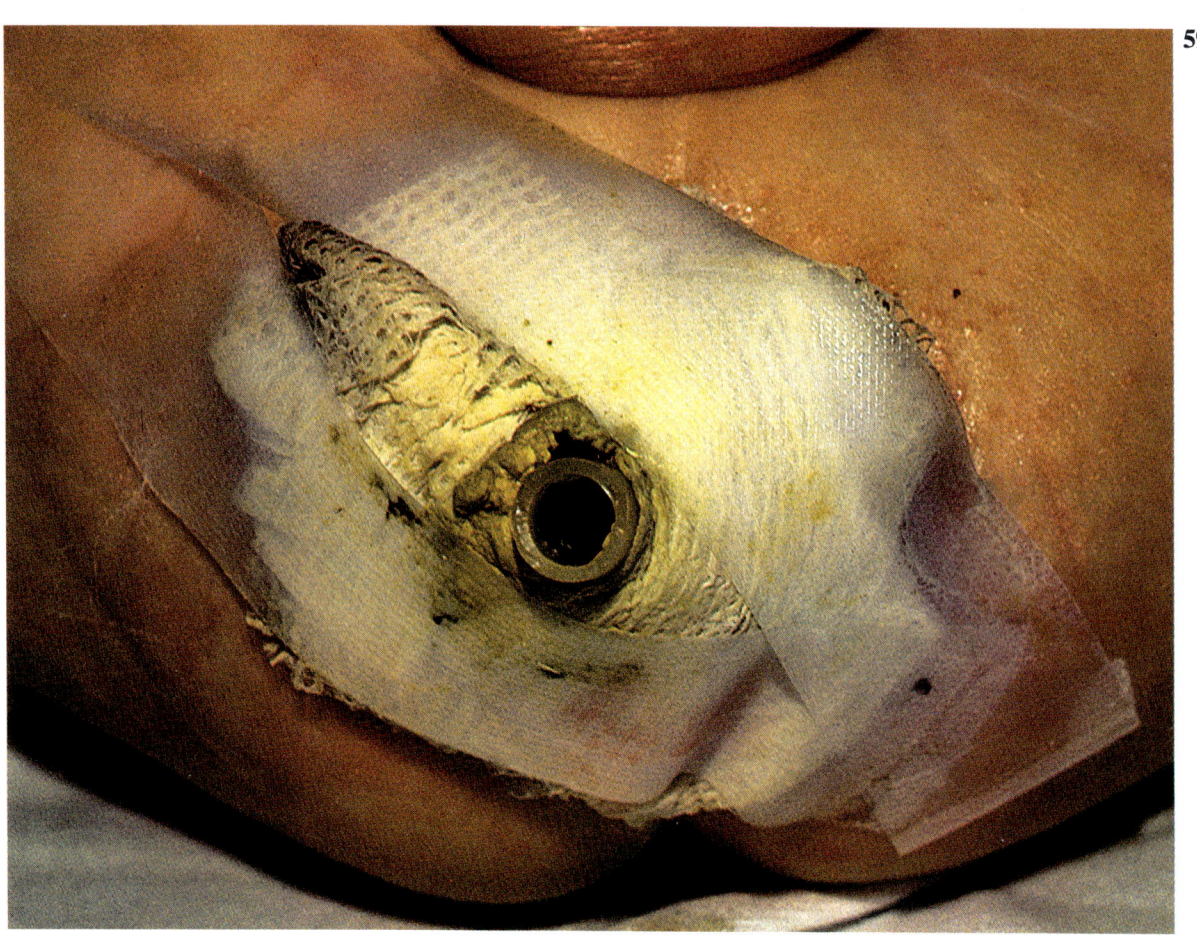

**59   A flatus tube is inserted into the rectum and a supporting tulle gras pack placed around the protruding colon.** It is kept clear by saline irrigation as needed to prevent any build-up in the rectum.

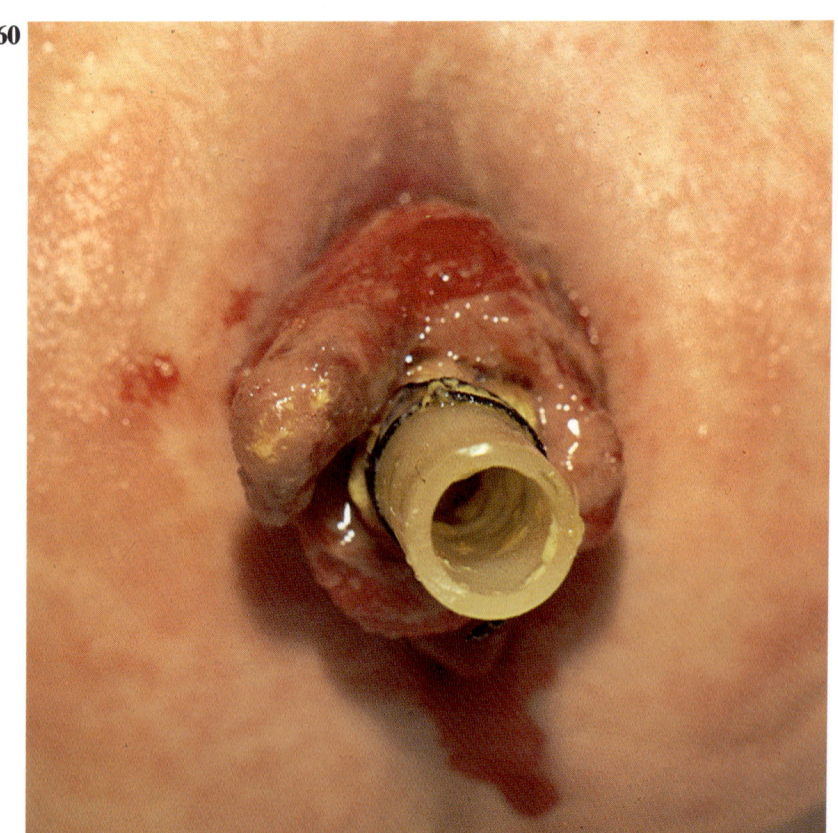

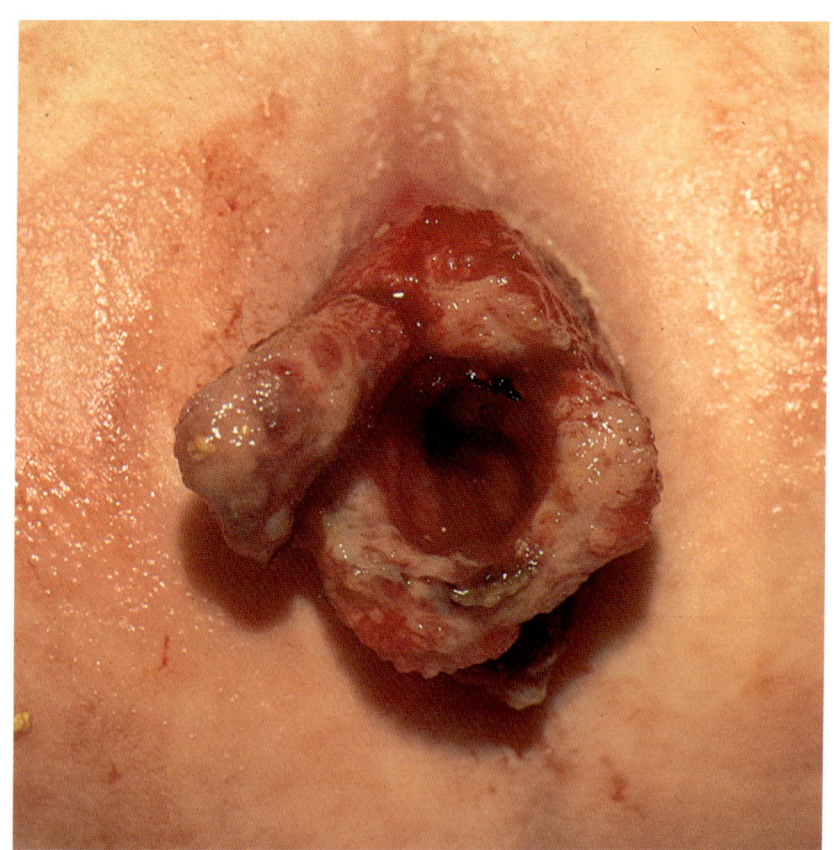

**60 and 61   The tube and dressing are removed in three or four days, because the tube may ulcerate the mucosa if left too long after tone has returned to the sphincter.** A flatus tube is passed as needed.

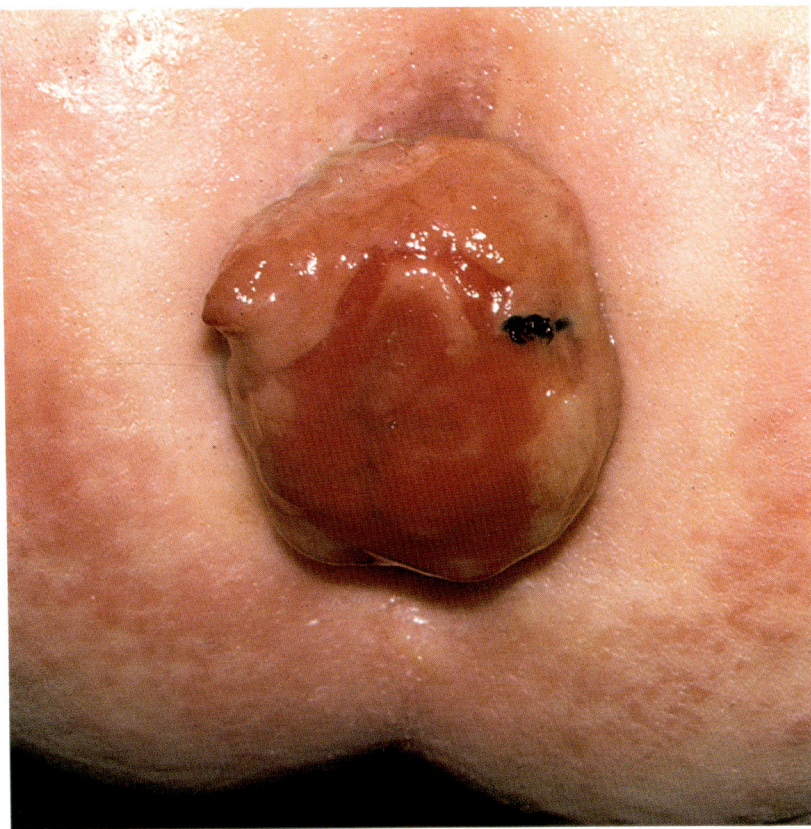

**62    At about 14 to 21 days the excess colon appears thus, and is ready for the completion operation.** If desired or convenient the child may have gone home with the 'anal colostomy' and may return later for the completion procedure.

**63    Traction on the colon demonstrates the level of adherence.** Half the circumference of the colon is divided and sutured to the everted anal canal.

A two-layer repair may be preferred and be more convenient if Soave's non-suture technique has been used, or the second layer is placed to complete the anastomosis if the author's preference for a staged procedure has been used.

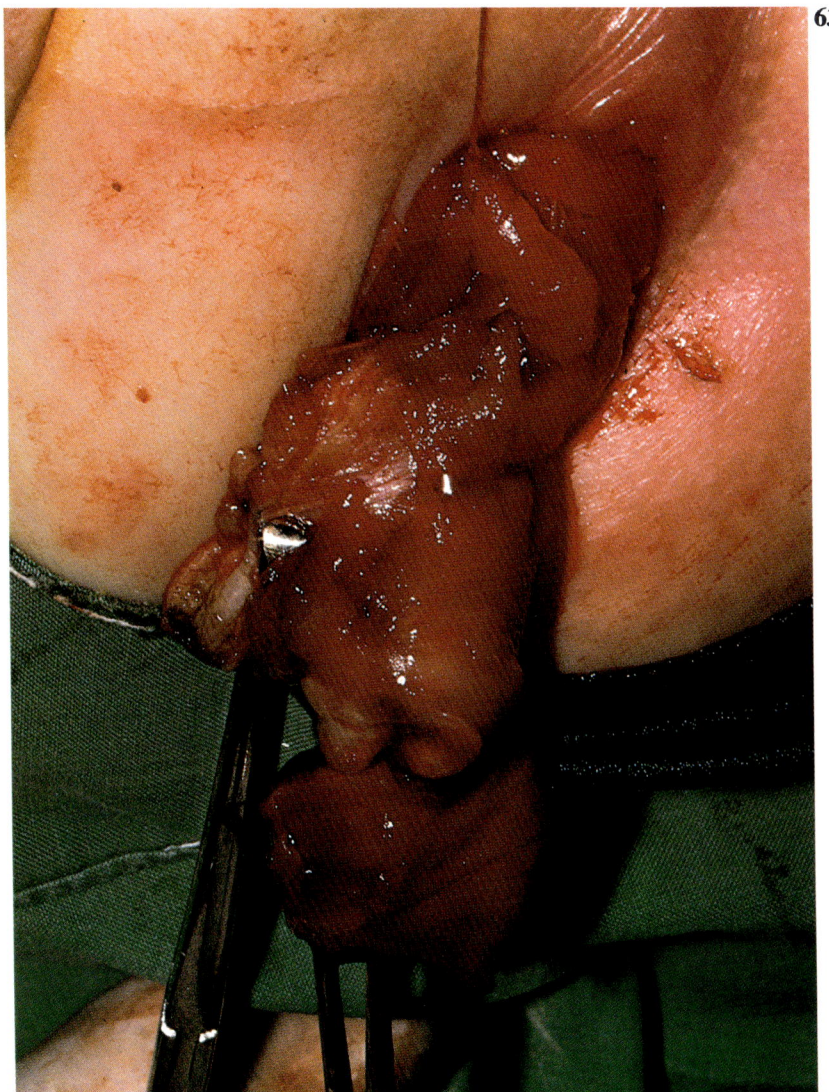

**64 Leaving two sutures long as retractors, the remainder of the circumference is divided and the anastomosis is completed.** Congestion sometimes makes this stage appear rather untidy but healing is sound, doubtless because of the good blood supply.

At this stage swelling makes the condition feel like a cervix uteri on rectal examination but does not interfere with function. However, fibrosis with healing may require one or more dilatations later. I first used this method in 1958, having heard Dr Ravitch's Hunterian Lecture on the 'Endorectal Technique for Colitis and Polyposis' given at the Royal College of Surgeons of England in 1949. At that time I had two suitable patients for a 'new' procedure who were to spend their lives in our care at Queen Mary's Hospital for Children, Carshalton. Because they progressed well for five years after operation, a further series was undertaken; these have progressed well for up to 20 years with normal control. My only reason for changing to other techniques was the need for postoperative dilatations, which could be distressing to the patients.

Because in my hands an experience of 400 patients still suggests that these other techniques require a covering colostomy for maximum protection from serious infective complications which, although uncommon, can endanger continence or even life, the choice of operation now becomes a matter of weighing one disadvantage against another.

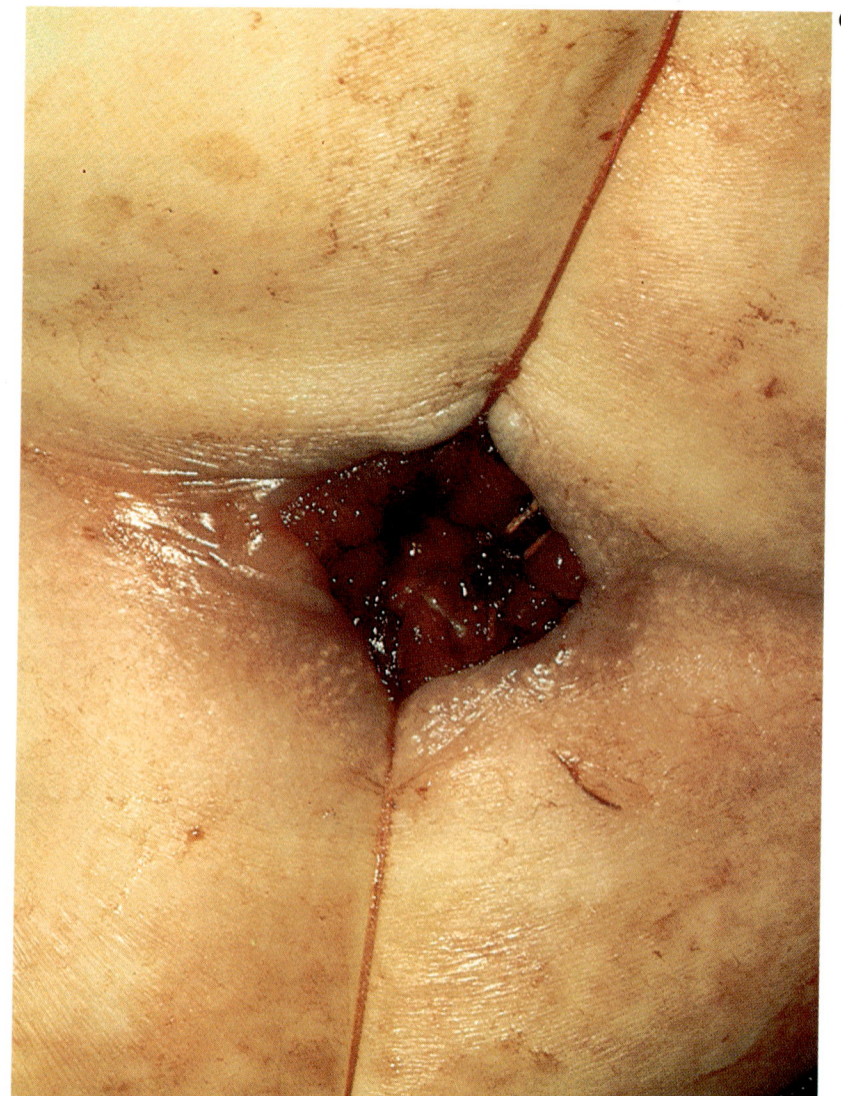

# Swenson prolapse procedure

**65   This is the same procedure up to 29** but division of terminal vessels on the exposed muscle coat of the rectum continues down to the anal canal at the level of the levators. This level can be assessed by a finger behind the rectum reaching far enough down to 'rock' the coccyx. Diathermy may be used for smaller vessels lower down but division between ligatures will still be needed for some vessels in spite of the dissection being on the muscle coat at the level where terminal vessels enter the bowel wall and **not** taking the lateral ligaments further from the rectum.

(This dissection may seem to go on for ever in older children, for the rectum is surprisingly misnamed. As its folds are liberated and it really becomes straight it seems to lengthen remarkably! It is crucial, nevertheless, that the dissection remains throughout on the muscle coat so as to avoid damage to the pelvic splanchnic nerves. Literally hundreds of cases, many now in married life, testify to the fact that when this technique is used there is no interference with urinary or sexual function.)

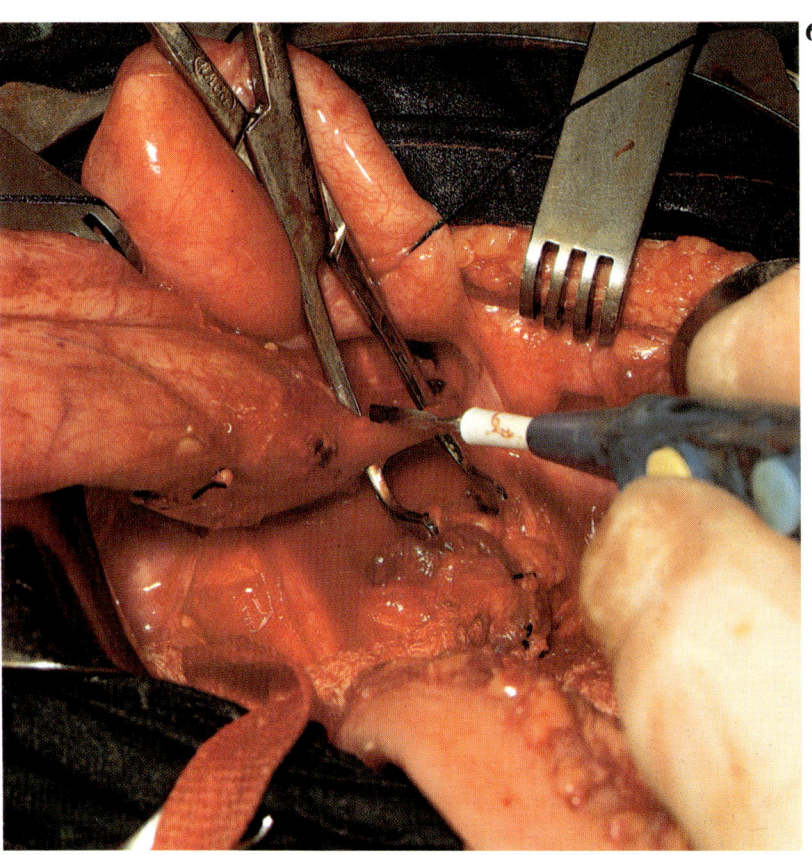

**66** **The bowel is divided at the upper end of the rectum and at the site confirmed for pullthrough by biopsy, and the intervening segment is discarded for histology in due course.** Division may be between clamps or by GIA stapler.

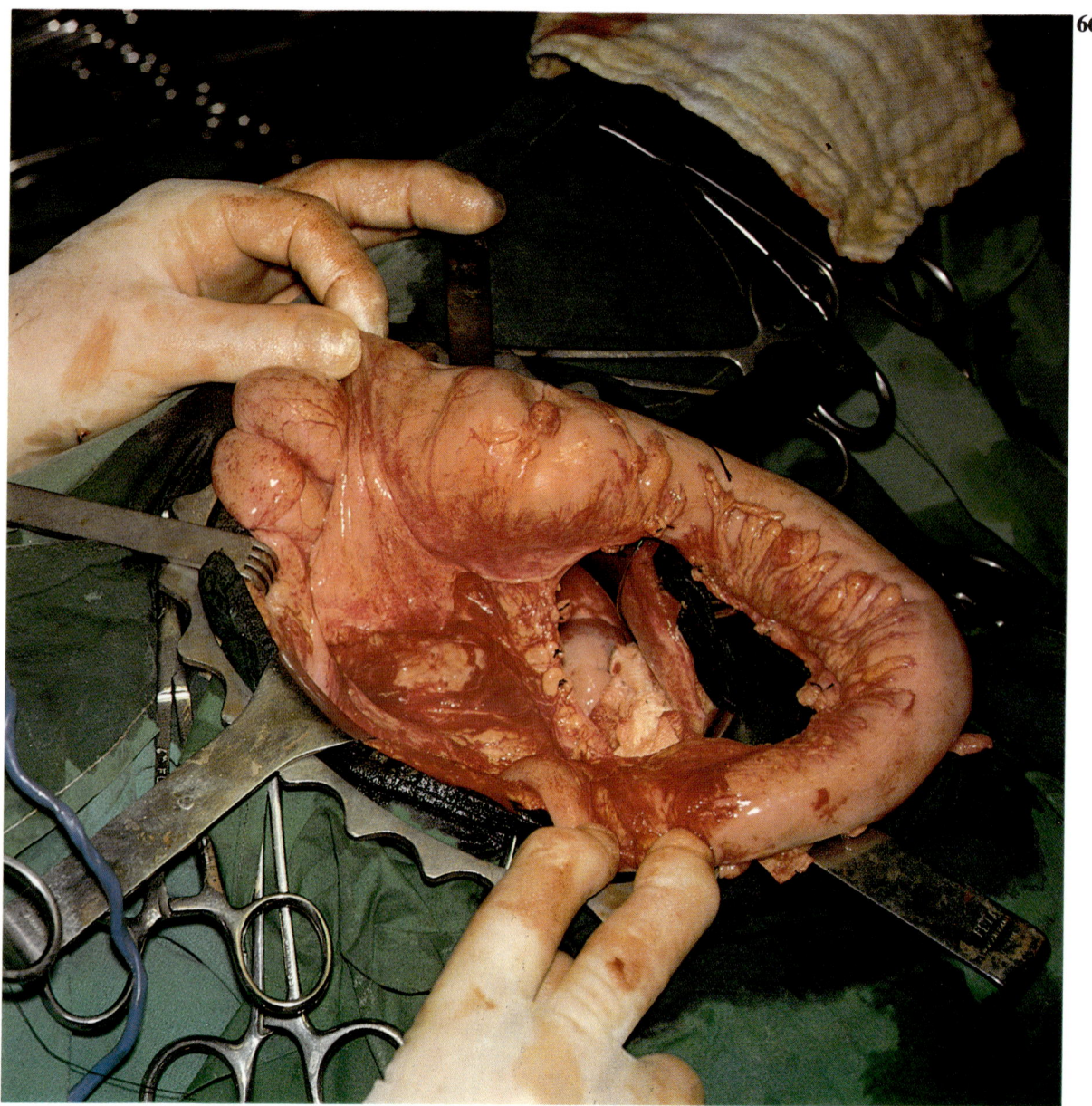

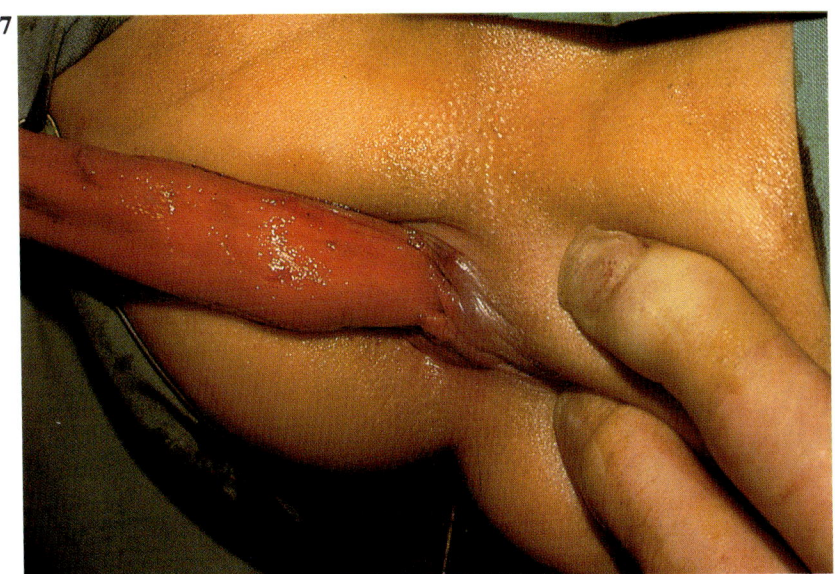

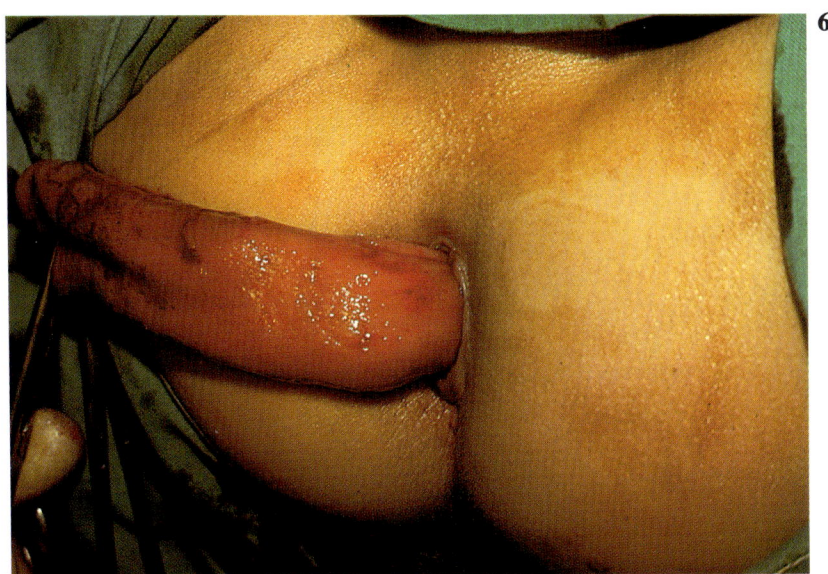

**67 and 68 The correct level of mobilisation is confirmed by prolapsing the rectum outside the anus.** It should be possible to unfold the sulcus by traction on the rectum but the anal canal should invert again spontaneously on releasing the tension.

**69 After povidone-iodine cleansing, one half of the everted rectum is opened.** The incision should begin anteriorly about 1 cm above the anal canal and descend posteriorly almost to reach the dentate line. (Hence the excision, when completed, should include an upper partial internal sphincterectomy.)

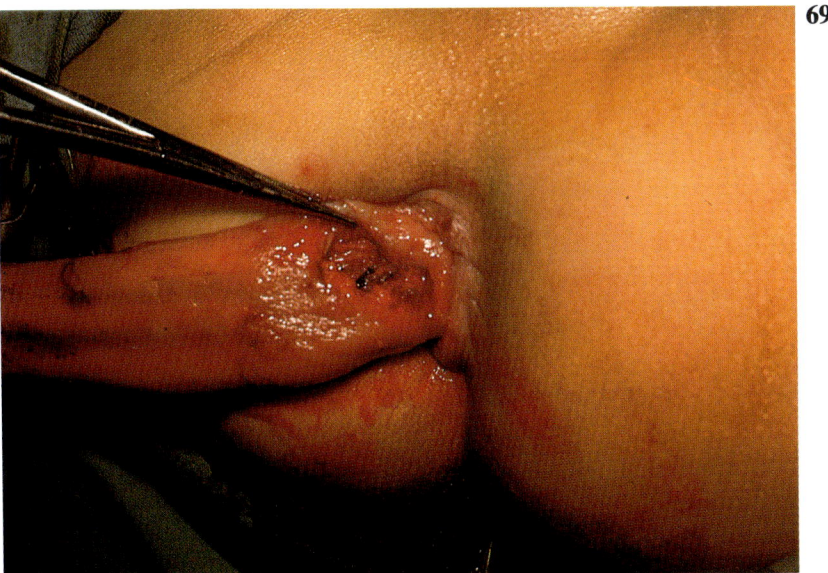

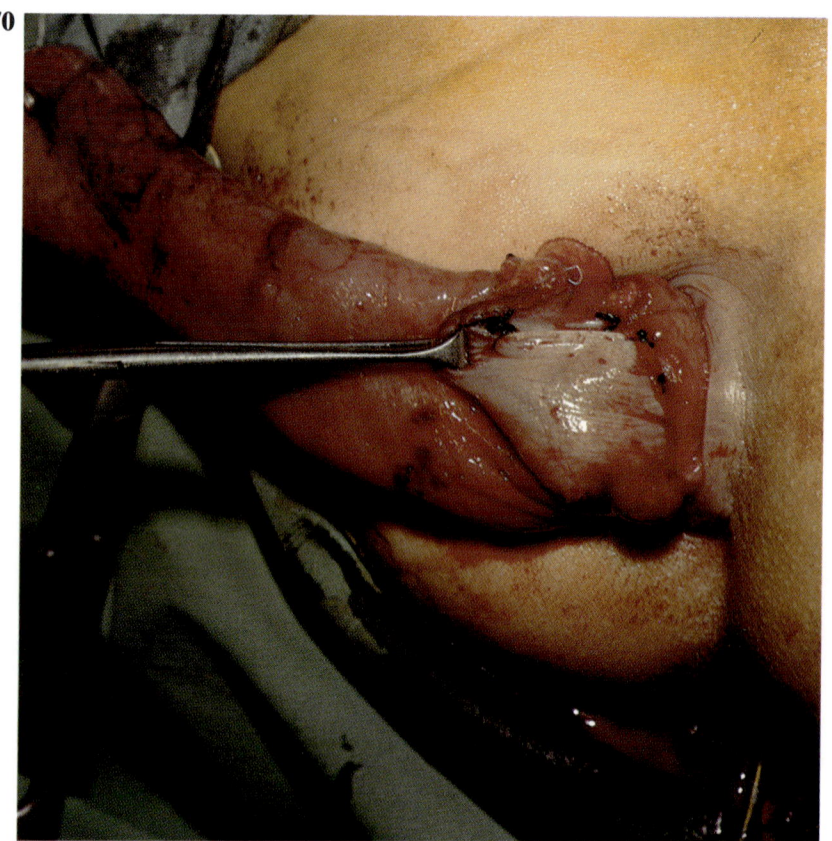 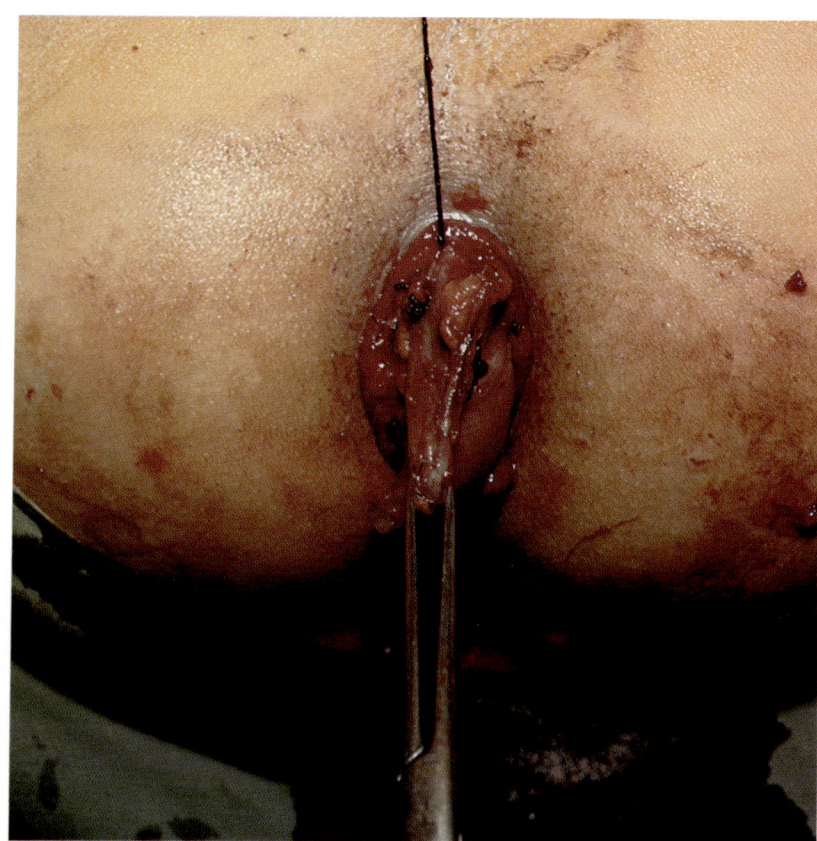

**70 and 71    A forceps is passed through the incision into the pelvis and the mobilised colon drawn down to the incision.** A layer of interrupted 4/0 or 3/0 Dexon or silk sutures is placed.

A similar incision is then made on the **opposite** side to complete the removal of the rectum and the layer of sutures is then completed.

**Note** Most authors describe the two-stage division of the rectum as an anterior half followed by the posterior half. I find it more convenient for the assistant, to do one side and then the other as illustrated here.

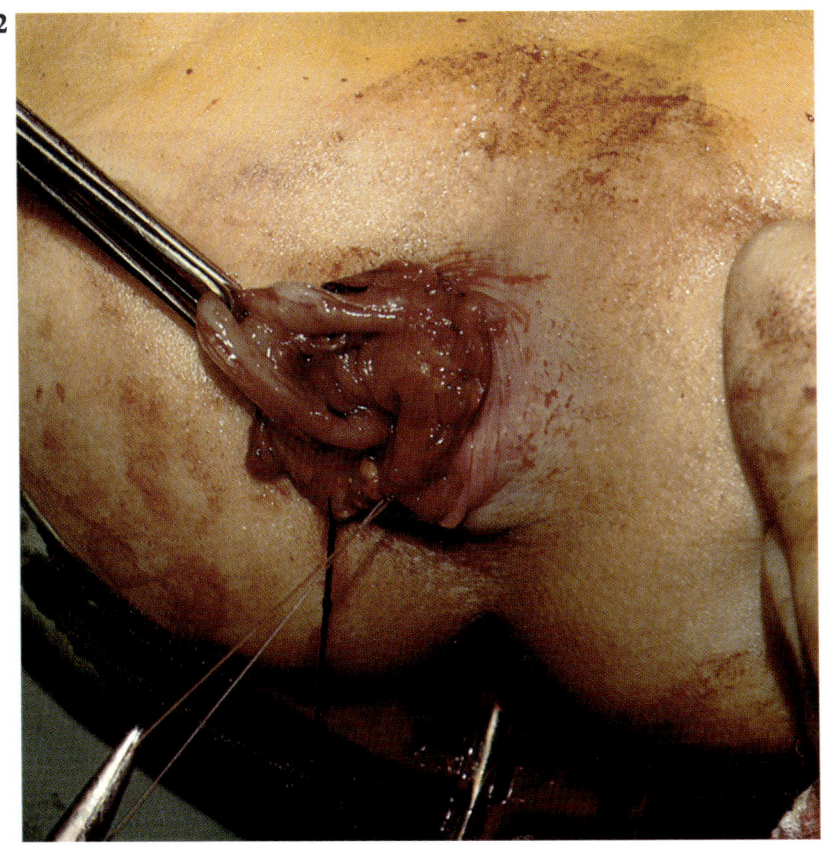

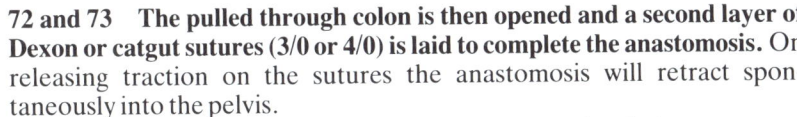

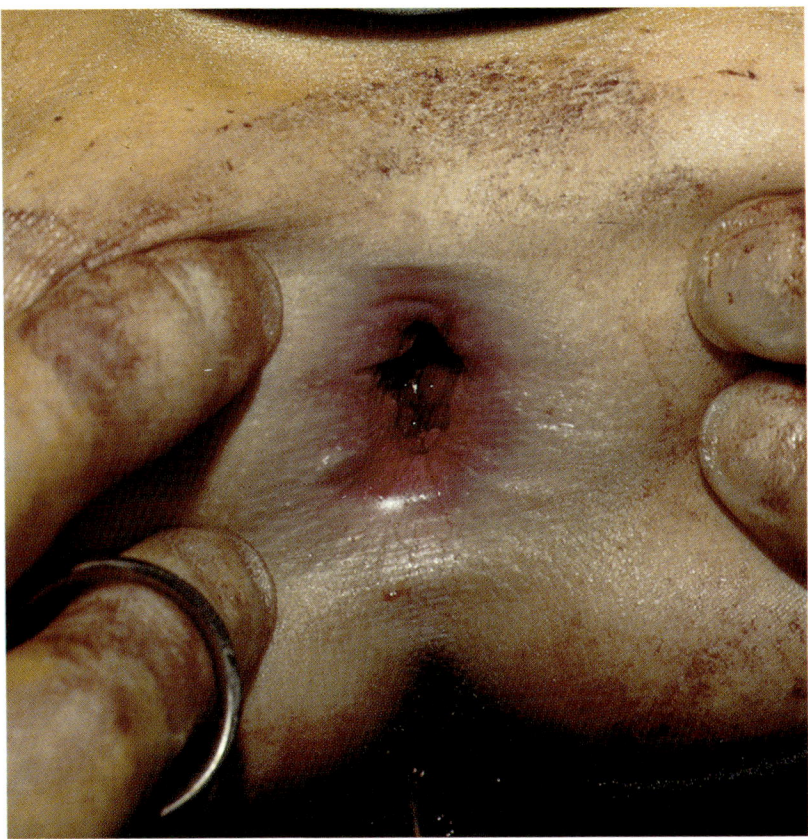

**72 and 73  The pulled through colon is then opened and a second layer of Dexon or catgut sutures (3/0 or 4/0) is laid to complete the anastomosis.** On releasing traction on the sutures the anastomosis will retract spontaneously into the pelvis.

Closure and drainage as described for the Duhamel technique.

Rectal digital examination is performed on the seventh postoperative day to confirm healing. If satisfactory, a contrast distal loop xray is undertaken. If there is no leak, the colostomy is closed 14 days after the original operation. If there is any leak – even a small and symptomless one – the child is sent out and a further xray made one month later. Although many of these radiological leaks may be insignificant, any fibrosis around the sphincters could interfere with fine continence. **I do not consider it justified to risk ignoring them.**

# Denis Browne's modification of the Swenson operation

**74 Sir Denis Browne's alternative method of performing the anal phase of the Swenson operation.**

The object is to avoid any opening or division of bowel within the abdomen.

The mobilised colon is intussuscepted out of the anus by traction on a heavy braided silk suture which has been looped around the rectosigmoid and threaded through the eye of a very long needle which is passed into the lumen of the bowel and down through a symoidoscope as a guide (**74**). The silk is snugged around the bowel at the tip of the sigmoidoscope. Light traction is then applied to the silk while the sigmoidoscope is withdrawn from the anus, prolapsing .the bowel out of the anus.

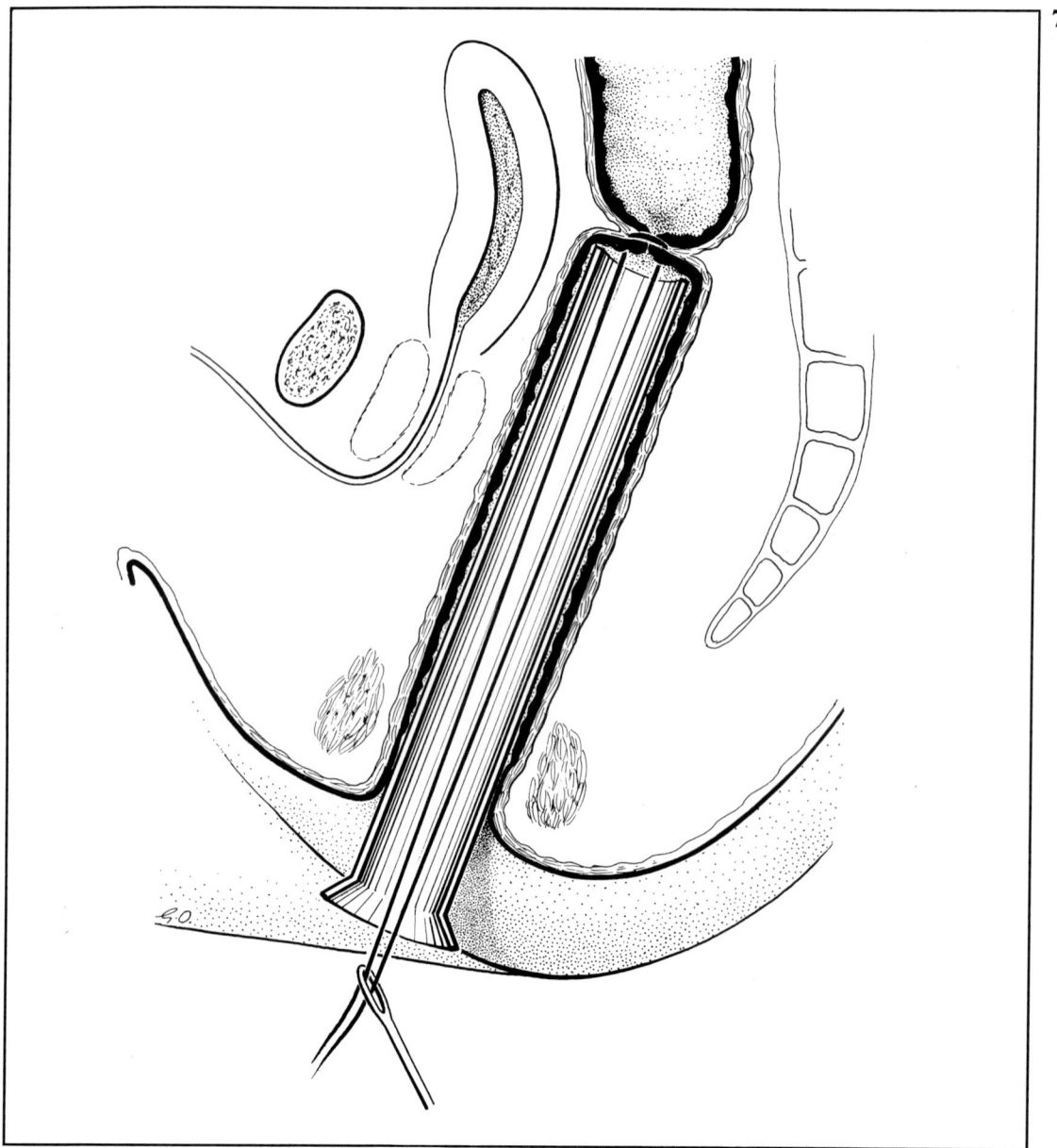

**75 Half the circumference of the rectum is divided at the upper end of the anal canal in the usual way.** The colon can then be intussuscepted unopened (unless very greatly enlarged – an uncommon occurrence now that cases are diagnosed earlier).

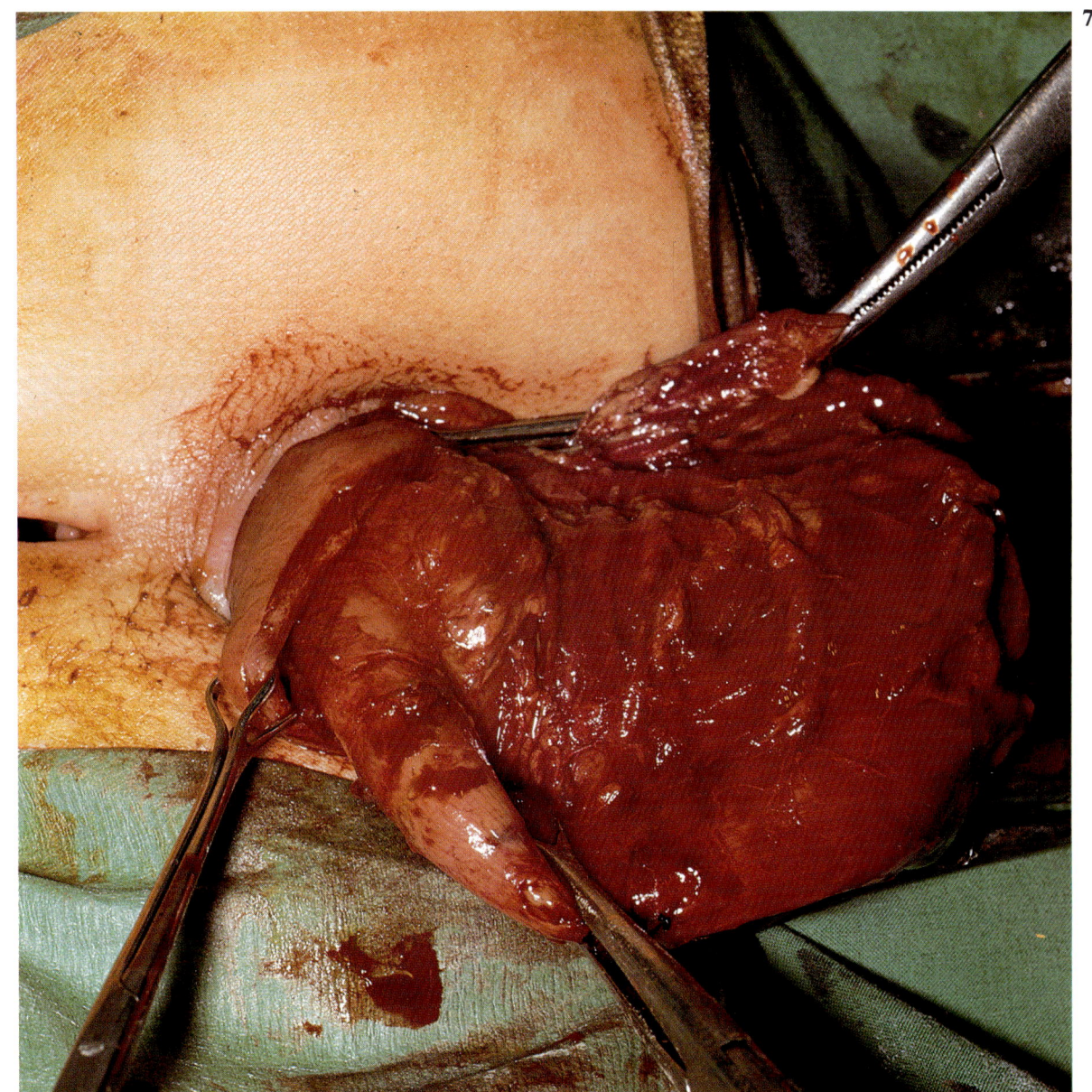

**76 to 78** The colon is then opened one quadrant at a time and four stay sutures are placed in turn and attached to the hooks of the 'suture plug' (**77**). This enables the assistant to control the bowel easily with one hand while the anastomosis is completed using the 'loop mattress suture'. The needle is passed from right to left for both insertions and the suture looped around the exiting needle point before drawing the needle out (**78**).

The suture plug is 'home made' of plastic (so that needles will not impact in it and diathermy can be used against it). Three sizes suffice from infant to adult.

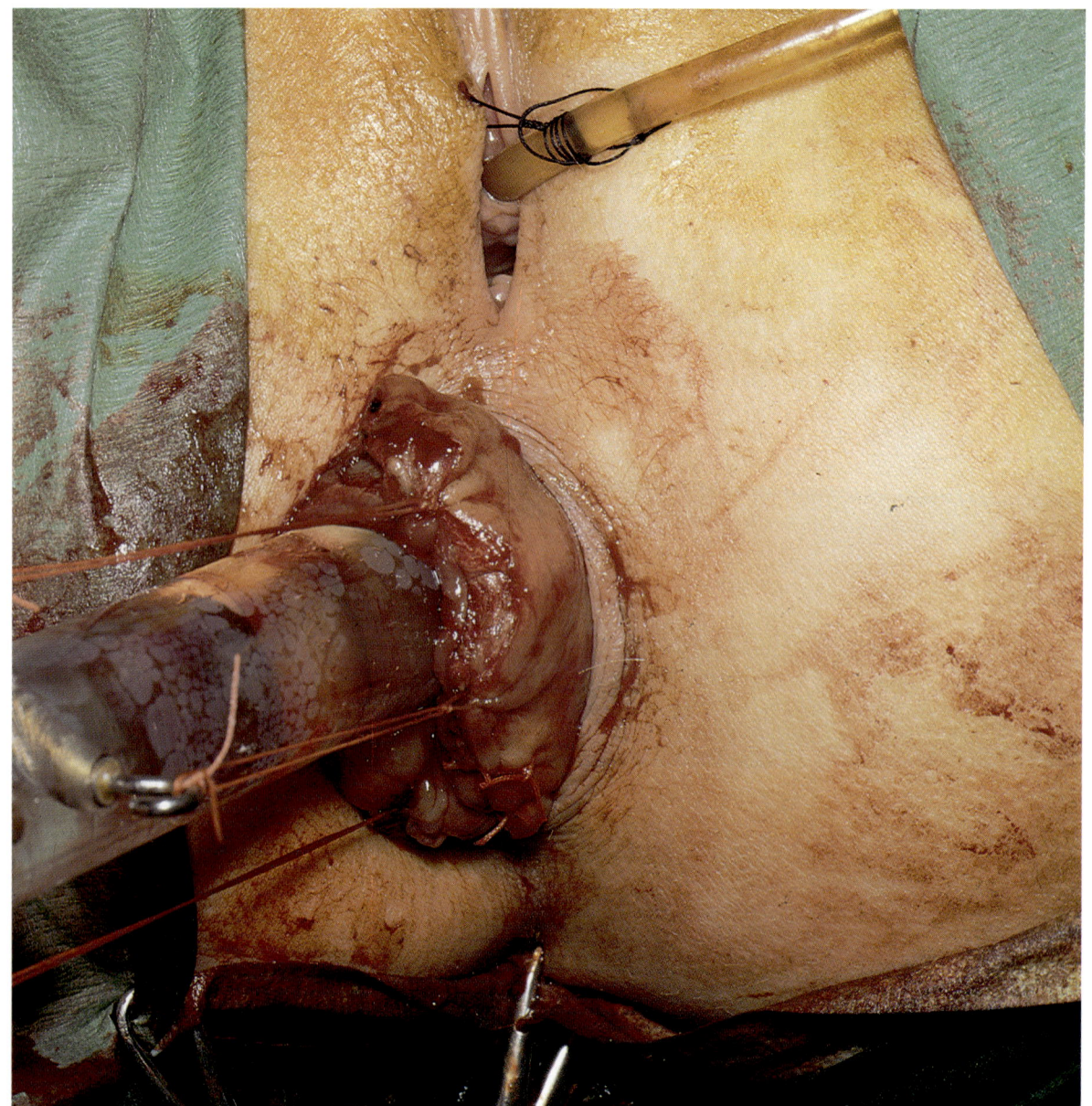

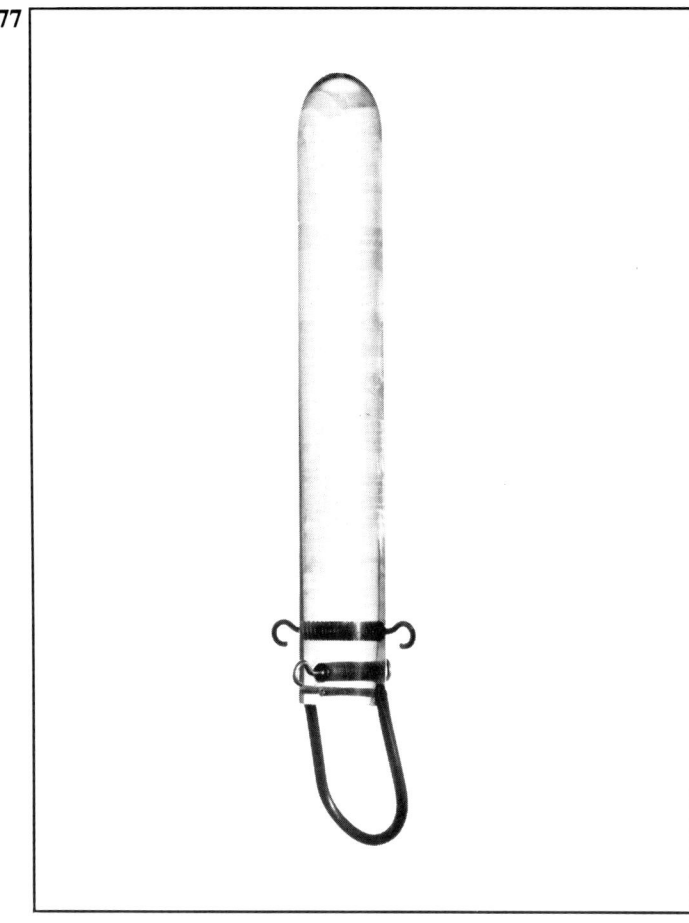

**77**

**78**

**78** The vertical mattress suture which apposes the mucosal edges as well as the muscle layers.

Suture looped around needle

Suture through eye

¾ Circle needle

Suture passing through bowel wall

Bowel wall

**77** The suture plug.

# References

1 Boley, S.J., 'Endorectal pullthrough operation with primary anasto-mosis for Hirschsprung's disease'. *Surg. Gynec. Obstet.* **127**, 353, 1968

2 Denda, T., 'Submucosal resection for Hirschsprung's disease'. *J. Jap. Assoc. Ped. Surg.* **6**, 189, 1970

3 Duhamel, B., 'A new operation for the treatment of Hirschsprung's disease'. *Arch. Dis. Childh.* **35**, 38, 1960

4 Frank, J.D. & Nixon, H.H., *Causes of death in Hirschsprung's disease. Analysis and Conclusions for Therapy in Progress in Pediatric Surgery*, Urban & Schwarzenberg, Philadelphia/Munich, Vol. 13 pp. 199–206, 1979

5 Hiatt, R.B., 'The surgical treatment of congenital megacolon'. *Ann. Surg.* **133**, 321, 1951

6 Khan, O. and Nixon, H.H., 'Results following surgery for Hirsch-sprung's disease: A review of three operations with a reference to neorectal capacity'. *Brit. J. Surg.* **67**, 436–438, 1980

7 Kimura, K., Nishijima, E., Muraji, T., Tsugasawa, C. and Matsumoto, Y., 'A new surgical approach to extensive aganglionosis'. *J. Pediat. Surg.* **16**, 840–843, 1981

8 Lake, B.D., Puri, P., Nixon, H.H. and Claireaux, A.E., 'Hirsch-sprung's disease. An appraisal of histochemically demonstrated acetylcholinesterase activity in suction rectal biopsy specimens as an aid to diagnosis'. *Arch. Path. Lab. Med.* **102**, 244–247, 1978

9 Lynn, H.B., 'Personal experience with rectal myectomy in the treatment of selected cases of aganglionic megacolon'. *Z. Kinderchir.* **5**, suppl. 98, 1968

10 Martin, L.W., 'Surgical management of total aganglionosis'. *Ann. Surg.* **176**, 343, 1972

11 Nixon, H.H., Colostomy. 'A simple technique and observations on indications.' *Z. Kinderchir.* **3**, 98–103, 1966

12 Nixon, H.H. and Lake, B.D., 'Not Hirschsprung's disease' – rare conditions with some similarities. *S. Afr. J. Surg.* **20**, 97–104, 1982

13 Noblett, H.R., 'A rectal suction biopsy tube for use in the diagnosis of Hirschsprung's disease'. *J. Pediat. Surg.* **4**, 406, 1969

14 Puri, P., Lake, B.D., Nixon, H.H., Mishalany, H. and Claireaux, A.E., 'Neuronal colonic dysplasia: An unusual association of Hirschsprung's disease'. *J. Pediat. Surg.* **12**, 681–685, 1977

15 Puri, P. & Nixon, H.H., 'Longterm results of Swenson's operation for Hirschsprung's disease' in *Progress in Pediatric Surgery*, Urban & Schwarzenberg, Philadelphia/Munich, Vol. **10**, pp. 87–96, 1977

16 Ravitch, M.M. and Sabiston, D.C. Jr., 'One stage resection of entire colon and rectum for ulcerative colitis and polypoid adenomatosis'. *Surg. Gynec. Obstet.* **84**, 1095, 1947

17 Rees, B.I., Azmy, A., Nigam, M. and Lake, B.D., 'Complications of rectal suction biopsy'. *J. Pediat. Surg.* **18**, 273–275, 1983

18 Rehbein, F. and Nicolai, I., 'Operative treatment for Hirschsprung's disease'. *German Med. Monthly,* **2**, 51–53, 1964

19 Soave, F., 'Hirschsprung's disease. Clinical evaluation and details of a personal technique'. *Z. Kinderchir.* suppl. 66, 1966

20 Swenson, O. and Bill, A.H., 'Resection of the rectum and recto-sigmoid with preservation of the sphincter for benign spastic lesions producing megacolon'. *Surgery,* **24**, 212, 1948

21 Swenson, O., 'Partial Internal Sphincterotomy in the treatment of Hirschsprung's disease'. *Ann. Surg.* **160**, 540, 1964

22 Thomas, D. F. M., Malone, M., Fernie, D. S., Bayston, R. and Spitz, L., 'Association between clostridium difficile and enterocolitis in Hirschsprung's disease'. *Lancet,* **i:** 78–79, 1982

# Further reading

*Hirschsprung's disease*, (Ed. A.M. Holschneider), Hippokrates Verlag, Stuttgart/Thieme-Stratton Inc, New York. (pp. 293, contributors 28), 1982

# Index

All figures are page numbers